Neuroendocrine Control of Metabolism

Editor

CHRISTOPH BUETTNER

ENDOCRINOLOGY AND METABOLISM CLINICS OF NORTH AMERICA

www.endo.theclinics.com

Consulting Editor
DEREK LEROITH

March 2013 • Volume 42 • Number 1

ELSEVIER

1600 John F. Kennedy Boulevard • Suite 1800 • Philadelphia, Pennsylvania, 19103-2899

http://www.theclinics.com

ENDOCRINOLOGY AND METABOLISM CLINICS OF NORTH AMERICA Volume 42, Number 1
March 2013 ISSN 0889-8529, ISBN-13: 978-1-4557-7084-7

Editor: Pamela Hetherington

Endocrinology and Metabolism Clinics of North America (ISSN 0889-8529) is published quarterly by Elsevier Inc., 360 Park Avenue South, New York, NY 10010-1710. Months of issue are March, June, September, and December. Periodicals postage paid at New York, NY and additional mailing offices. Subscription prices are USD 313.00 per year for US individuals, USD 557.00 per year for US institutions, USD 159.00 per year for US students and residents, USD 393.00 per year for Canadian individuals, USD 681.00 per year for Canadian institutions, USD 456.00 per year for international individuals, USD 681.00 per year for international institutions, and USD 234.00 per year for international and Canadian and foreign students/residents. To receive student/resident rate, orders must be accompanied by name of affiliated institution, date of term, and the signature of program/residency coordinator on institution letterhead. Orders will be billed at individual rate until proof of status is received. Foreign air speed delivery is included in all *Clinics* subscription prices. All prices are subject to change without notice. **POSTMASTER:** Send address changes to *Endocrinology and Metabolism Clinics of North America*, Elsevier Health Sciences Division, Subscription Customer Service, 3251 Riverport Lane, Maryland Heights, MO 63043. **Customer Service: Telephone: 1-800-654-2452** (U.S. and Canada); **1-314-447-8871** (outside U.S. and Canada). **Fax: 1-314-447-8029. E-mail: journalscustomerservice-usa@elsevier.com** (for print support); **journalsonlinesupport-usa@elsevier.com** (for online support).

Reprints. For copies of 100 or more, of articles in this publication, please contact the Commercial Rights Department, Elsevier Inc., 360 Park Avenue South, New York, NY 10010-1710; phone: (+1) 212-633-3813; fax: (+1) 212-462-1935; e-mail: reprints@elsevier.com.

Endocrinology and Metabolism Clinics of North America is covered in *MEDLINE/PubMed (Index Medicus)*, *EMBASE/Excerpta Medica, Current Contents/Clinical Medicine, Current Contents/Life Sciences, Science Citation Index, ISI/BIOMED, BIOSIS,* and *Chemical Abstracts.*

Printed and bound by CPI Group (UK) Ltd, Croydon, CR0 4YY

Transferred to digital print 2012

Contributors

CONSULTING EDITOR

DEREK LEROITH, MD, PhD
Chief, Division of Endocrinology, Metabolism and Bone Diseases, Department of Medicine, Mount Sinai School of Medicine, New York, New York

EDITOR

CHRISTOPH BUETTNER, MD, PhD
Departments of Medicine and Neuroscience, Mount Sinai School of Medicine, New York, New York

AUTHORS

JENS C. BRÜNING, MD
Department of Mouse Genetics and Metabolism, Institute for Genetics, Center for Endocrinology, Diabetes and Preventive Medicine (CEDP), University Hospital Cologne and Center for Molecular Medicine Cologne (CMMC), University of Cologne; Cologne Excellence Cluster on Cellular Stress Responses in Aging Associated Diseases (CECAD); Max-Planck-Institute for Neurological Research, Köln, Germany

ALEJANDRO CAICEDO, PhD
Diabetes Research Institute; Program in Neuroscience, Departments of Medicine, Physiology and Biophysics, Miller School of Medicine, University of Miami, Miami, Florida

AMY L. CLARK, DO
Division of Endocrinology and Diabetes, Department of Pediatrics, Washington University, St Louis, Missouri

PENNY DACKS, PhD
Aging & Alzheimer's Disease Prevention, Alzheimer's Drug Discovery Foundation, New York, New York

MARK L. EVANS, MD
Metabolic Research Laboratories, Department of Medicine, Institute of Metabolic Science, University of Cambridge, Cambridge, United Kingdom

SIMON J. FISHER, MD, PhD
Associate Professor of Medicine, Cell Biology and Physiology, Division of Endocrinology, Metabolism and Lipid Research, Departments of Medicine, Cell Biology and Physiology, Washington University, St Louis, Missouri

CRISTINA GARCÍA-CÁCERES, PhD
Institute for Diabetes and Obesity, Helmholtz Centre Munich, Garching, Munich, Germany

MANFRED HALLSCHMID, PhD
Department of Medical Psychology and Behavioral Neurobiology, University of Tuebingen; Institute for Diabetes Research and Metabolic Diseases of the Helmholtz Centre Munich, University of Tuebingen (Paul Langerhans Institute Tuebingen), Tuebingen, Germany

JOERG HEEREN, PhD
Department of Biochemistry and Molecular Cell Biology, University Medical Center Hamburg-Eppendorf, Hamburg, Germany

FUMIKO ISODA, PhD
Department of Neuroscience, Mount Sinai School of Medicine, New York, New York

HENDRIK LEHNERT, MD
Department of Internal Medicine I, University of Luebeck, Luebeck, Germany

MARINA LITVIN, MD
Division of Endocrinology, Metabolism and Lipid Research, Department of Medicine, Washington University, St Louis, Missouri

CHARLES V. MOBBS, PhD
Department of Neuroscience, Mount Sinai School of Medicine, New York, New York

CESAR MORENO, BA, BS
Department of Neuroscience, Mount Sinai School of Medicine, New York, New York

HEIKE MÜNZBERG, PhD
Department of Central Leptin Signaling, Pennington Biomedical Research Center, LSU Systems, Baton Rouge, Louisiana

MAYOWA A. OSUNDIJI, PhD
Metabolic Research Laboratories, Department of Medicine, Institute of Metabolic Science, University of Cambridge, Cambridge, United Kingdom

MICHAEL POPLAWSKI, MD, PhD
Department of Neuroscience, Mount Sinai School of Medicine, New York, New York

CANDACE M. RENO, PhD
Division of Endocrinology, Metabolism and Lipid Research, Department of Medicine, Washington University, St Louis, Missouri

RAYNER RODRIGUEZ-DIAZ, PhD
Diabetes Research Institute, Miller School of Medicine, University of Miami, Miami, Florida

MARIANNA SADAGURSKI, PhD
Department of Endocrinology, Children's Hospital Boston, Howard Hughes Medical Institute, Boston, Massachusetts

THOMAS SCHERER, MD
Division of Endocrinology and Metabolism, Department of Internal Medicine III, Medical University of Vienna, Vienna, Austria

GARY J. SCHWARTZ, PhD
Departments of Medicine and Neuroscience, Diabetes Research and Training Center, Bronx, New York

SOPHIE M. STECULORUM, PhD
Department of Mouse Genetics and Metabolism, Institute for Genetics, Center for
Endocrinology, Diabetes and Preventive Medicine (CEDP), University Hospital Cologne
and Center for Molecular Medicine Cologne (CMMC), University of Cologne; Cologne
Excellence Cluster on Cellular Stress Responses in Aging Associated Diseases (CECAD);
Max-Planck-Institute for Neurological Research, Köln, Germany

MATTHIAS H. TSCHÖP, MD
Division of Metabolic Diseases, Department of Medicine, Technical University Munich,
Munich, Germany; Institute for Diabetes and Obesity, Helmholtz Centre Munich;
Institute for Diabetes and Obesity, Business Campus Garching-Hochbrück, Garching,
Munich, Germany

MERLY C. VOGT
Department of Mouse Genetics and Metabolism, Institute for Genetics, Center for
Endocrinology, Diabetes and Preventive Medicine (CEDP), University Hospital Cologne
and Center for Molecular Medicine Cologne (CMMC), University of Cologne; Cologne
Excellence Cluster on Cellular Stress Responses in Aging Associated Diseases (CECAD);
Max-Planck-Institute for Neurological Research, Köln, Germany

MORRIS F. WHITE, PhD
Department of Endocrinology, Children's Hospital Boston, Howard Hughes Medical
Institute, Boston, Massachusetts

LINDA YANG, PhD
Beth Israel Deaconess Medical Center, Harvard Medical School, Boston, Massachusetts

CHUN-XIA YI, MD, PhD
Institute for Diabetes and Obesity, Helmholtz Centre Munich, Garching, Munich, Germany

Contents

> Islet hormones, especially insulin and glucagon, are important for glucose homeostasis. Insulin is a necessity for life, and disturbed insulin release results in disordered blood glucose regulation. Although isolated islets are fully capable of detecting changes in their local environment (particularly glucose fluctuations) and altering hormone release appropriately, experimentally manipulating pancreatic innervation alters islet hormone release in the whole animal. This article describes how brain may play a role in influencing and directing secretion of insulin and glucagon as a key part of the integrated physiology of blood glucose homeostasis.

> For people with diabetes, hypoglycemia remains the limiting factor in achieving glycemic control. This article reviews recent advances in how the brain senses and responds to hypoglycemia. Novel mechanisms by which individuals with insulin-treated diabetes develop hypoglycemia unawareness and impaired counterregulatory responses are outlined. Prevention strategies for reducing the incidence of hypoglycemia are discussed.

> The autonomic nervous system helps regulate glucose homeostasis by acting on pancreatic islets of Langerhans. Despite decades of research on the innervation of the pancreatic islet, the mechanisms used by the autonomic nervous input to influence islet cell biology have not been elucidated. This article discusses how these barriers can be overcome to study the role of the autonomic innervation of the pancreatic islet in glucose metabolism. It describes recent advances in microscopy and novel approaches to studying the effects of nervous input that may help clarify how autonomic axons regulate islet biology.

Obesity is characterized by a chronic and low-grade inflammation in tissues including the hypothalamus. Hypothalamic inflammation is considered an early and determining factor for the onset of obesity, a factor that occurs even before body weight gain. Within the hypothalamus, microglia and astrocytes produce cytokines that drive inflammatory responses. Astrocytes are directly affected by nutrient excess and might play a unique role in promoting hypothalamic inflammatory responses in obesity. This article reviews evidence supporting the role of hypothalamic astrocytes in obesity, and suggests a new approach for neuroendocrine research designed to reveal pathogenesis and develop novel treatment strategies against obesity.

All organisms must adapt to changing nutrient availability, with nutrient surplus promoting glucose metabolism and nutrient deficit promoting alternative fuels (in mammals, mainly free fatty acids). A major function of glucose-sensing neurons in the hypothalamus is to regulate blood glucose. When these neurons sense glucose levels are too low, they activate robust counterregulatory responses to enhance glucose production, primarily from liver, and reduce peripheral metabolism. Some hypothalamic neurons can metabolize free fatty acids via β-oxidation, and β-oxidation generally opposes effects of glucose on hypothalamic neurons. Thus hypothalamic β-oxidation promotes obese phenotypes, including enhanced hepatic glucose output.

This article reviews recent studies identifying two key brain regions as two critical nodes in the neural network where central leucine sensing contributes to whole body energy homeostasis: the mediobasal hypothalamus and the dorsal vagal complex of the caudal brainstem. Activation of these leucine sensing sites engages multiple determinants of energy balance, including glucose homeostasis, food intake, and adiposity.

During the last decades, obesity research has focused on food intake regulation, whereas energy expenditure has been mainly measured based on whole-body oxygen consumption. With the renaissance of brown adipose tissue (BAT) thermogenesis as a potential drug target in humans, more thought is put into alternative heat-producing mechanisms. Also, the interaction of peripheral and central components to regulate thermogenesis requires further studies. Certainly, several of the novel molecular genetic tools available now, compared with 40 years ago, will be helpful to gain new insights in BAT-controlled energy homeostasis and promises new approaches to pharmacologically control body weight.

Besides the well-characterized effects of brain insulin and leptin in regulating food intake, insulin and leptin signaling to the central nervous system modulates a variety of metabolic processes, such as glucose and lipid homeostasis, as well as energy expenditure. This review summarizes the current literature on the contribution of central nervous insulin and leptin action to metabolic control in animals and humans. Potential therapeutic options based on the direct delivery of these peptides to the brain by, for example, intranasal administration, are discussed.

The insulin pathway coordinates growth, development, metabolic homoeostasis, fertility, and stress resistance, which influence life span. Compensatory hyperinsulinemia to overcome systemic insulin resistance circumvents the immediate consequences of hyperglycemia. Work on flies, nematodes, and mice indicate that excess insulin signaling damages cellular function and accelerates aging. Maintenance of the central nervous system (CNS) has particular importance for life span. Reduced insulin/IGF1 signaling in the CNS can dysregulate peripheral energy homeostasis and metabolism, promote obesity, and extend life span. Genetic manipulations of insulin/IGF1 signaling components are revealing neuronal circuits that might resolve the central regulation of systemic metabolism from organism longevity.

It is increasingly accepted that the metabolic future of an individual can be programmed as early as at developmental stages. For instance, offspring of diabetic mothers have a greater risk of becoming obese and diabetic later in life. Animal studies have demonstrated that hyperinsulinemia and/or hyperglycemia during perinatal life permanently impair the organization and long-term function of hypothalamic networks that control appetite and glucose homeostasis. This review summarizes the main findings regarding the key regulatory roles of perinatal insulin and glucose levels on hypothalamic development and on long-term programming of metabolic diseases reported in different rodent models.

ENDOCRINOLOGY AND METABOLISM CLINICS OF NORTH AMERICA

RELATED INTEREST

Endocrinology Clinics, Volume 41, Issue 2 (June 2012)
Insulin-Like Growth Factors in Health and Disease
Claire M. Perks and Jeff M.P. Holly, *Editors*

NOW AVAILABLE FOR YOUR iPhone and iPad

Foreword

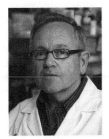

Derek LeRoith, MD, PhD
Consulting Editor

This issue covers an emerging issue, namely, the central control of metabolism. Until recently, it was believed that control of peripheral metabolism was that peripheral tissue's response to nutrients and hormonal control was directly on the tissue itself, and only appetite and satiety were controlled by the hypothalamus. We now have evidence to the contrary; control of peripheral metabolism is both central and peripheral.

As described by Drs Osundiji and Evans, pancreatic release of insulin and glucagon is regulated at the local level as well as centrally. They describe many of these central control mechanisms, including direct autonomic neural efferents, both sympathetic and parasympathetic, and detail the nuclei in the brain that control these pathways. They further describe the effect of glucose and lipids on the hypothalamic control of pancreatic hormone release as well as central GLP-1 effects, the role of the melanocortin system. Finally, in regard to hypothalamic effects of glucagon release secondary to hypoglycemia, there are a number of mechanisms being researched including K/ATP channels, AMPK activity, and glucose transport changes.

Hypoglycemia remains a major obstacle to patients with diabetes and health care providers attempting to improve metabolic control. Glucagon and the sympathetic nervous system response are the main counterregulatory hormonal responses in the acute setting of hypoglycemia, and the central nervous system responds to low glucose levels, leading to the patient's awareness of the critical fall in blood glucose. In their article, Drs Reno, Litvin, Clark, and Fisher discuss hypothalamic centers, such as the VMH and arcuate nucleus, that are responsive to low glucose levels. The VMH, for example, activates the sympathetic nervous system peripherally. In addition, extra hypothalamic centers are activated. Most importantly is their description of the potential mechanisms that affect the counterregulatory effects and lead to hypoglycemic unawareness. They describe CRF, cortisol, opioids, and sleep effects as blunting the response in addition to the effect of repeated hypoglycemia leading to alterations in cellular glucose uptake and metabolism in hypothalamic areas.

All in all, the research in this area is critical to our understanding and avoidance of hypoglycemia and hypoglycemia unawareness.

It has become commonly accepted that the autonomic nervous system regulates glucose homeostasis. As described in their article, Drs Rodriquez-Diaz and Caicedo

Endocrinol Metab Clin N Am 42 (2013) xi–xiii
http://dx.doi.org/10.1016/j.ecl.2012.12.002
0889-8529/13/$ – see front matter © 2013 Published by Elsevier Inc.

explain that the autonomic innervation of the β cells of the islets has been established; however, the exact mechanism of how autonomic innervation regulates islet cell biology is yet to be well defined. Both sympathetic and parasympathetic nerves are found in the islets and apparently release neurotransmitters, such as acetylcholine and noradrenaline, that then act on receptors on the various islet cells. In addition, neuropeptides, such as VIP, NPY, and galanin, are released and have effects on the β and α cells. Parasympathetic innervation enhances secretion, whereas sympathetic innervation generally inhibits secretion. Recent reports have suggested that eliminating pancreatic sensory innervation may affect the immune response in models of type 1 diabetes and add to defective insulin secretion in models of type 2 diabetes. The authors discuss the difficulties in establishing the exact mechanisms involved in these overall processes and suggest that integrative histologic and in vivo studies may help better define the mechanisms involved in normal control of islet function by the nervous system and the abnormality that occurs in disease states.

Body weight is clearly regulated by the hypothalamus, because numerous signals regulate energy expediture and energy balance in addition to suppressing appetite and thermogenesis. In models of obesity, there is evidence of hypothalamic resistance not only to the action of insulin and leptin but also to certain cytokines. Drs García-Cáceres, Yi, and Tschöp posit that hypothalamic astrocytes, which are sensitive to nutrient intake, signal the hypothalamic nuclei, inducing the cytokine resistance. The evidence, of course, is derived from animal models, but the idea is compelling and suggests an area of research worth pursuing in the search for therapies for obesity.

The focus of the article by Drs Moreno, Yang, Dacks, Isoda, Poplawski, and Mobbs is on hypothalamic adaptation to nutrient availability. They describe how hypothalamic neurons not only sense changes in glucose levels, thereby regulating counterregulatory hormonal effects, but are also capable of robust metabolizing of free fatty acids (FFAs), such as octanoate and palmitic acid by β-oxidation. This effect counteracts glucose effects on these neurons and has been invoked in resultant obesity and hyperglycemia. This central effect of FFAs is apparently mediated by alterations in expression and/or activity of PPAR-α, although this effect is not fully defined.

Nutrient signaling in the brain has focused primarily on glucose and free fatty acids. Dr Schwartz discusses in his article that amino acids such as leucine may also have important signaling effects through the mediobasal hypothalamus and the dorsal vagal complex of the caudal brainstem. These effects are via the mTOR-S6 kinase pathway, similar to the effects of amino acids on peripheral tissues. The importance of these findings is that leucine signaling can protect against HFD-induced obesity because it causes an increase in energy expenditure via these central effects. The implications of this for our obesity epidemic may be very significant.

One of the hot topics in adipose tissue biology and physiology is the "browning of fat." As Drs Heeren and Münzberg describe, brown fat (BAT) is involved in dissipating excess energy by generating heat, whereas white adipocytes (WAT) store triglycerides and are known to release adipokines. There are a number of factors that regulate WAT conversion to BAT as well as BAT activity. These include cold, exercise, diet, and aging as well as thyroid hormones, to name but a few important ones. Given its effects on energy balance, researchers are now trying to determine how BAT activity can be harnessed to treat obesity and diabetes.

In their article on insulin and leptin effects on the brain, Drs Scherer, Lehnert, and Hallschmid review the studies showing that both hormones feedback to inhibit appetite. In addition, they both regulate peripheral metabolism, energy expenditure, and energy balance. Most recently, evidence is developing that they have other properties such as memory formation and emotions, and insulin in particular has been implicated in the pathophysiology of Alzheimers and other neurodegenerative disorders. The authors suggest that both hormones may have potential for future therapeutics in regard to their action on the brain.

When the insulin/IGF-1 signaling system in primitive organisms such as *Caenorhabditis elegans* and *Drosophila melanogaster* is inhibited, lifespan is extended, as it has been similarly demonstrated in rodents. As Drs. Sadagurski and White discuss, the question arises as to whether this is a feature of insulin resistance or reduced insulin signaling, especially because the former has negative implications, whereas the latter may be associated with caloric restriction that positively impacts longevity. They discuss insulin signaling in the periphery and in the brain and present evidence from multiple rodent models that have reduced growth hormone, IGF-1, or insulin levels and are associated with longevity. In particular, they discuss the effect of the brain insulin/IGF-1 system and neurodegenerative disorders: work from their own studies. They hypothesize that the brain signaling pathways may play an important role in longevity; we anxiously await further definitive data on this important issue.

The role of epigenetics and imprinting in generational effects of the metabolic syndrome and type 2 diabetes have become an important area of investigation. It potentially explains how the offspring of diabetic mothers are prone to develop metabolic diseases. Drs Steculorum, Vogt, and Brüning propose that the abnormality in metabolism such as hyperglycemia may alter insulin signaling in the developing hypothalamus. Their suggestions are derived from experimental evidence whereby HFD feeding may alter hypothalamic neurocircuit development. Although this area of research needs more investigation, it may partially explain the increased metabolic syndrome of the offspring exposed to the maternal environment.

Dr Buettner and his colleagues have achieved a phenomenal result. They have contributed articles that describe the basic science behind the central control of metabolism and feeding behavior as well as response to hypoglycemia, and they have made it extremely readable to all of us and of practical importance. We owe them our gratitude.

Derek LeRoith, MD, PhD
Division of Endocrinology, Metabolism, and Bone Diseases
Department of Medicine
Mount Sinai School of Medicine
One Gustave L. Levy Place
Box 1055, Altran 4-36
New York, NY 10029, USA

E-mail address:
derek.leroith@mssm.edu

Preface

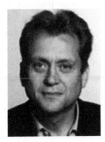

Christoph Buettner, MD, PhD
Editor

As we are faced with an epidemic of obesity and type 2 diabetes of historic dimensions, we continue to strive to understand the pathophysiology of both of these conditions. A field that offers important insights into the link between overnutrition and obesity and diabetes is the neuroendocrinology of metabolism and energy homeostasis. Progress in this area has been impressive over the last 2 decades and the field continues to expand, making it difficult for a broader readership to keep abreast. This becomes all the more relevant with the recent advent of diabetes drugs that work predominantly or in part via the central nervous system (CNS), such as cycloset (bromocriptine) or GLP1 agonists, respectively. The aim of this edition of *Endocrinology and Metabolism Clinics of North America* is to highlight new aspects of neuroendocrine regulation that are of fundamental biological or clinical relevance. I have selected colleagues that are at the front of their fields to review these emerging areas of studies and I have enjoyed reading their insightful reviews.

It is now well established that the CNS plays a central role in appetite regulation, but also in regulating systemic carbohydrate and lipid metabolism. Nutrients, such as glucose and amino acids, and hormones, such as insulin and leptin, are sensed by the brain and these indicators of nutrient availability are integrated with neuronal signals from the periphery to fine-tune systemic nutrient partitioning and hormone secretion in peripheral organs like liver, pancreas, and adipose tissue. A relatively underexplored area is how the brain regulates hormonal secretion in the endocrine pancreas and in what way the autonomic nervous system controls hormone secretion, specifically, in human islets. The brain is central in maintaining euglycemia, not at least to warrant its own survival as no other organ depends as exclusively on glucose as fuel as the brain. There are several reviews in this edition that highlight novel aspects of how central nutrient and hormone sensing regulates glucose homeostasis. Based on these insights, intranasal delivery of insulin or leptin, which in principle is a way to deliver peptides to the brain, has the potential to emerge as antidiabetic or antiobesity drugs, which is one of several innovative therapeutic strategies that are covered within this volume of *Endocrinology and Metabolism Clinics of North America*.

There is clearly a link between metabolic dysregulation and inflammation, although the causal relationship is still a matter of controversy. Obesity and diabetes are also

Endocrinol Metab Clin N Am 42 (2013) xv–xvi
http://dx.doi.org/10.1016/j.ecl.2013.01.001
0889-8529/13/$ – see front matter © 2013 Published by Elsevier Inc.

endo.theclinics.com

associated with inflammation in the hypothalamus, which has the potential to impair CNS control of metabolism. Brown adipose tissue has recently reemerged as a promising area for investigation for two reasons, first due to its unique thermogenic capacity, that, when activated, can markedly increase energy expenditure, and, second, because a series of reports have established its presence in humans, which was doubted just a few years ago. Last and somewhat philosophically are the provocative reviews into the role of CNS insulin and leptin signaling during intrauterine development as a key metabolic programming pathway that can be a feed-forward mechanism explaining why children of obese mothers face increased metabolic risk, and finally, how hypothalamic insulin and IGF1 signaling may regulate lifespan.

Thus, in summary, I believe this edition brings us up to date in these interesting fields and will stimulate clinical reasoning.

Christoph Buettner, MD, PhD
Departments of Medicine and Neuroscience
Mount Sinai School of Medicine
One Gustave L. Levy Place
New York, NY 10029, USA

E-mail address:
christoph.buettner@mssm.edu

Brain Control of Insulin and Glucagon Secretion

Mayowa A. Osundiji, PhD, Mark L. Evans, MD*

KEYWORDS

- Glucose stimulated insulin secretion • Autonomic control of pancreas
- Hypoglycemia • Islets of langerhans • Hypothalamus • Glucose sensing • Insulin
- Glucagon

KEY POINTS

- The pancreas is innervated by both parasympathetic and sympathetic nervous systems and both exocrine and endocrine pancreatic secretion can be altered by activity in neural inputs to pancreas.
- For both insulin and glucagon, it seems likely that brain acting via neural control facilitates local islet responses as part of the integrated homeostatic control of blood glucose levels.
- The relative importance of local and neural factors in release of insulin and glucagon in response to changes or threatened changes in blood glucose remain to be fully determined.

INTRODUCTION

The islets of Langerhans are heavily involved in glucose homeostasis, releasing insulin and glucagon into the portal circulation to influence glucose balance. Integrated release of insulin and glucagon from islets is carefully controlled, and although there is no doubt that islets are fully capable of independent insulin and glucagon release, the pancreas is richly innervated, and several studies have shown that neural influences can alter islet hormone release.[1–3] Increasingly, an important contribution from brain in controlling other aspects of glucose homeostasis is being described. For example, several studies have suggested that the basomedial hypothalamus controls hepatic glucose balance via vagal efferents (eg, Ref.[4]), sensing locally changes in nutrients and with brain perhaps acting also as a site for insulin action (see article by Scherer elsewhere in this issue).

The integrated control of insulin release is of obvious relevance for those interested in diabetes and metabolic disease. In addition, a better understanding of glucagon release is of particular topical interest, given the current resurgence of interest in

Neither author has any relevant disclosures or conflicts of interest.

Metabolic Research Laboratories, Department of Medicine, Institute of Metabolic Science, University of Cambridge, Box 289, Addenbrooke's Hospital, Hills Road, Cambridge CB2 0QQ, UK
* Corresponding author.
E-mail address: mle24@cam.ac.uk

how disturbances in glucagon may contribute to the pathophysiology of diabetes. Hyperglucagonemia as an adverse cause in type 2 diabetes has long been postulated.[5] Recent data examining glucagon receptor null mice show that loss of glucagon action protects against ketoacidosis, suggesting that, in the presence of insulinopenia, a relative hyperglucagonemia may contribute to the metabolic disturbances seen in type 1 diabetes.[6] In addition, loss of glucagon responses to hypoglycemia is a major part of the abnormal counterregulation that leads to the increased risk of hypoglycemia in type 1 and some patients with type 2 diabetes and is covered in depth by a separate review by Fisher elsewhere in this issue.

In this review, the evidence for the role of brain in modulating islet secretion is presented, focusing on glucagon and insulin release from the pancreas.

PANCREATIC INNERVATION

To influence pancreatic islet secretion, the brain needs to exert control either directly by innervation or indirectly by altering circulating factors affecting islet activity. In this section, the innervation of the pancreas is described and the effects of direct autonomic neural efferents on islet secretion are summarized. A more comprehensive review of pancreatic innervation is available in the article by Caicedo elsewhere in this issue. The pancreas is richly innervated by both sympathetic (splanchnic) and parasympathetic (vagus) systems. Stimulation of the vagus increases pancreatic insulin output,[1,2,7] whereas the net effect of splanchnic nerve stimulation is to reduce insulin and increase glucagon output.[3,8]

Parasympathetic preganglionic fibers innervating the pancreas emanate from the dorsal motor nucleus of the vagus as part of the bulbar outflow tract,[9] arriving via the hepatic and gastric vagal branches to synapse at intrapancreatic ganglia, from which postganglionic nerves pass to islets. In general, vagal stimulation stimulates secretion of insulin, glucagon, somatostatin, and pancreatic polypeptide, the latter sometimes being used as a marker of pancreatic vagal activity.[10] Vagal activity probably acts through acetylcholine actions on muscarinic M_3 receptor in both α and β cells to stimulate glucagon and insulin secretion, respectively.[11–13] However, there may be additional parasympathetic actions through noncholinergic neurotransmitters such as the neuropeptides vasoactive intestinal polypeptide (VIP), pituitary adenylate cyclase-activating polypeptide (PACAP), and gastrin-releasing peptide (GRP). VIP, PACAP, and GRP are found in islet parasympathetic terminals and act to stimulate insulin release.[14,15]

For sympathetic innervation, preganglionic fibers originate from C8 to L3 spinal cord outflow, running via the lesser and greater splanchnic nerves to synapse in the paravertebral ganglia or celiac ganglion. Postganglionic noradrenergic fibers then enter the pancreas, although some preganglionic fibers may also reach islets. In general, sympathetic stimulation increases glucagon and decreases insulin and somatostatin secretion.[16] Noradrenaline released from sympathetic terminals has differing effects on different islet cell types. In α cells, α_2 and β_2 adrenoreceptors act to increase glucagon release. In contrast, α_2 receptors in β cells are coupled via Gi-mediated signaling to reduce glucose-stimulated insulin secretion, the dominant effect of sympathetic activation on β cells.[17] However, pancreatic β cells also contain β_2 adrenoreceptors, which can stimulate insulin release. As for the parasympathetic system, nonclassic neurotransmitters (in this case, galanin and neuropeptide Y) are found and may also influence islet secretion.[18]

Nonautonomic pancreatic innervation has also been identified. For example, islets may have neural connections with sensory nerves, nitric oxide neurons, and local enteric neurones as part of a local enteric circuit.[19] The relative importance of all of these inputs in controlling islet secretion is uncertain. In general, it is likely that neural input from brain interacts with other circulating and local factors to control islet secretion in an integrated fashion.

CENTRAL BRAIN CONNECTIONS TO PANCREAS

Central brain connections of the pancreas can be examined by using retrograde tracers such as pseudorabies virus injected into the pancreas. In a comprehensive study by Jansen and colleagues[20] using this approach, 1 group of rats underwent ablation of celiac ganglia and sympathetic innervation so that pancreatic injection of pseudorabies labeled the central parasympathetic connections. A second group underwent subdiaphragmatic vagotomy, allowing the central sympathetic connections to be visualized.

There were important overlaps and some distinct differences between the 2 autonomic systems. For the parasympathetic connections, brain stem labeling was seen (as anticipated) in dorsal vagal nucleus and in the nucleus tractus solitarius, area postrema, and paratrigeminal nuclei. Other areas with virally infected cells included the dorsal paragigantocellular nucleus, rostral ventrolateral medulla, lateral paragigantocellular reticular nucleus, raphe magnus, and gigantocellular reticular nucleus. Labeling was also seen in the midbrain (ventrolateral part of the periaqueductal gray) and pons (A5 and subcoeruleus regions). In the hypothalamus, virally infected parasympathetic preganglionic neurons were seen in the paraventricular nucleus (parvicellular portion), dorsomedial nucleus and in the dorsal and lateral (perifornical and caudal lateral) hypothalamus. Infected cells were also seen in the central nucleus of amygdala and the bed nucleus of the stria terminalis.

For sympathetic connections, cell body labeling was found in the rostral ventrolateral medulla, lateral paragigantocellular reticular nucleus, and gigantocellular reticular nucleus. Infected neurons were also localized in the caudal raphe nuclei (raphe obscurus, pallidus, and magnus). Outside the brain stem, labeling was seen in the cervical spinal cord, midbrain (periaqueductal gray and Edinger-Westphal nucleus) pons (A5 region, locus coeruleus, subcoeruleus nucleus, and Barrington nucleus) and medial preoptic area. In the hypothalamus, labeling was seen in the paraventricular nucleus (parvicellular part), lateral hypothalamic area (perifornical and caudal regions), and dorsal hypothalamus.

Although this study and similar approaches cannot distinguish between exocrine and endocrine pancreatic connections, other data also suggest that some of the areas listed earlier are important in controlling endocrine pancreatic secretion. Some nuclei with overlapping sympathetic and parasympathetic connections have also been identified as being associated with sympathoadrenal preganglionic neurones, suggesting that these areas might be involved in the central maintenance of glucose homeostasis.[21,22] Further evidence for a hypothalamic role is presented later. For the brain stem, chemical stimulation of the dorsal vagal complex or connected raphe obscurus nucleus increases islet secretion.[23,24]

BRAIN NUTRIENT SENSING AND INSULIN SECRETION

Brain contains specialized nutrient sensors capable of detecting changes in glucose and other nutrients and responding by triggering energy and glucose homeostatic responses. Several studies have examined whether brain nutrient sensing can affect insulin secretion. In a series of studies, Penicaud's group have shown that a small glucose bolus given directly into rat carotid artery directed toward brain can rapidly induce a peripheral insulin secretory response. The amount of glucose administered was not enough to result in a detectable increase in systemic blood glucose, suggesting that effects were attributable to local brain detection of an increase in glucose. Insulin secretion was associated with activation of neurones in the paraventricular nucleus and activation of both neurones and astrocytes in the arcuate nucleus of the hypothalamus. The insulin secretory response to intracarotid glucose delivery was abolished by the astrocyte poison methionine sulfoximine, suggesting that glial cells in the arcuate nucleus are a critical part of this reponse.[25] In subsequent in vivo and ex vivo studies, the same group suggested that glucose detection occurs by the transient generation of reactive oxygen species by the glucose load, a type of redox signaling.[26]

Penicaud's group have also examined how fatty acids may alter insulin secretion via the brain. Intracerebroventricular (ICV) infusion of intralipid and heparin for 48 hours in rats led to enhanced insulin secretion during a conventional intravenous glucose tolerance test (IVGTT). However, blood glucose values after the glucose challenge were similar, suggesting reduced insulin sensitivity. Insulin clamp studies confirmed that the brain lipid infusion also resulted in hepatic insulin resistance, so that it is unclear whether the increased insulin secretion was a direct effect on pancreas or not. In support of a direct effect, brain lipid infusion also led to reduced pancreatic noradrenaline turnover, suggesting that reduced pancreatic sympathetic activity might be underpinning the changes.[27] A follow-up study showed a similar effect with intracarotid lipid infusion, which could be blocked with etomoxir, an inhibitor of β-oxidation, suggesting that metabolism of lipid was necessary for effects to be seen. In keeping with hypothalamic mediation, intracarotid lipid infusion was associated with reduced activation in several nuclei implicated in nutrient sensing or autonomic control (arcuate, dorsomedial, paraventricular, and ventromedial nuclei), but with increased activation in the lateral hypothalamus. These changes in activation were all reversed by etomoxir.[28]

We recently examined how hypothalamic glucose sensing might integrate with peripheral islet glucose sensing, performing IVGTTs in rats. Delivery of a small amount of glucose direct into the third ventricle boosted early phase insulin secretory responses and reduced the excursion in plasma glucose (**Fig. 1**). These data suggested that brain areas around the third ventricle were capable of sensing the change in glucose and triggering an amplification of insulin secretory responses. We hypothesized that the detection of a change of glucose might use the low-affinity hexokinase, glucokinase (GK), analogous to the mechanisms used in the pancreatic β cell. To test this hypothesis, we performed intravenous glucose challenges in animals in the presence of GK inhibitors, glucosamine, or mannoheptulose. Central GK inhibition reduced the insulin secretory response and increased systemic glucose excursions after the glucose bolus.[29]

Lesioning studies of the basomedial hypothalamus, although a crude approach, also support a hypothalamic role in modulating glucose-stimulated insulin release, with insulin secretion being reduced 10 minutes after an electrolytic lesioning of the area of the ventromedial hypothalamus (VMH) in anesthetized rats.[30] Other data also suggest that hypothalamic areas have a central controlling role in insulin secretion in response to neuropeptides. Knockdown of insulin receptors in the VMH area using an antisense vector resulted in impaired glucose-induced insulin secretion during hyperglycemic clamps studies. In addition, there were paradoxic rises in glucagon during ramped hyperinsulinemic euglycemia, suggesting that hypothalamic insulin signaling is important in directing integrated islet responses.[31] Glucagonlike peptide 1 (GLP-1) is a powerful stimulus acting direct at the β cell to amplify glucose-stimulated insulin secretion. GLP-1 also has brain effects to alter energy and glucose homeostasis. Knauf and colleagues[32] showed that ICV brain infusion of exendin 4,

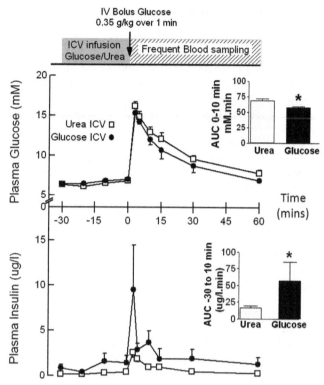

Fig. 1. Brain delivery of glucose increases insulin secretion in response to a glucose challenge. Chronically catheterized male Sprague-Dawley rats underwent 30-minute ICV delivery of 9 mg glucose or an osmotic control (urea) followed by an IVGTT (0.35 g/kg glucose in urea-treated rats with dose reduced by 9 mg in glucose-infused rats so that the same total glucose dose was delivered into the body). (*Top panel*) ICV glucose-infused rats showed improved glucose handling during the first 10 minutes of the IVGTT, with a significantly lower area under the curve (AUC0–10) relative to urea-infused animals (*top panel inset*). (*Lower panel*) Plasma insulin levels in ICV glucose-infused rats were significantly higher than controls with insulin secretion between the start of the brain infusion and the 10-minute time point of the IVGTT (cutoff between early and late phase insulin secretion) was significantly higher in ICV glucose-infused rats (*lower panel inset*). *$P<.05$. (*Data from* Osundiji MA, Lam DD, Shaw J, et al. Brain glucose sensors play a significant role in the regulation of pancreatic glucose-stimulated insulin secretion. Diabetes 2012;61(2):321–8.)

a GLP-1 agonist, increased insulin secretion in response to hyperglycemia induced by intravenous insulin infusion. When glucose was delivered intragastrically, a route likely to induce significant GLP-1 release, brain delivery of exendin 9 (a GLP-1 antagonist) reduced insulin secretory responses.

Together, these studies suggest that brain glucose sensors, probably located in key nuclei in the hypothalamus, play a role in the control of insulin secretion, at least in early phase responses after a glucose challenge. The magnitude of the contribution of brain glucose sensors in the regulation of insulin release in these experiments was modest relative to direct β-cell pathways. Overall, the studies are suggestive of a model whereby an increase in blood glucose level is detected by specialized brain sensors in addition to direct sensing by pancreatic β cells, to facilitate glucose-stimulated insulin secretion.

If the hypothalamus does play a role in controlling glucose-stimulated insulin secretion, particularly early phase, could hypothalamic changes underpin the loss of insulin secretion that occurs as type 2 diabetes develops? Loss of early phase insulin secretion is a key feature as individuals progress from being insulin-resistant (but able to compensate through increased insulin release) to impaired glucose tolerance/frank diabetes. A recent report has examined the role of hypothalamic inflammation in this process. Rats fed a high-fat diet developed impaired first-phase insulin release in response to a glucose load similar to the changes seen in humans. This loss of first-phase insulin release was paralleled by hypothalamic inflammation. In high-fat-fed rats, first-phase insulin secretion was improved by sympathectomy or brain delivery of infliximab, an antitumor necrosis factor α (anti-TNF-α) therapy. In chow-fed rats, high-fat-dietlike effects on early phase insulin secretion were mimicked by brain delivery of TNF-α.[33] Thus, not only might hypothalamus have a role in controlling physiology of insulin release but it might also be involved in the pathophysiologic process whereby high-fat feeding or obesity lead to dysfunctional insulin secretion and diabetes.

BRAIN MELANOCORTIN SYSTEM AND INSULIN SECRETION

In recent years, the melanocortin system has emerged as a key controller in determining many aspects of energy and nutrient homeostasis. Evidence has now emerged that brain melanocortin signaling is involved in the central control of insulin secretion: (1) ICV administration of the melanocortin 3 receptor or melanocortin 4 receptor (MC4R) agonist, melanotan II, in mice decreased insulin level[34]; (2) ICV leptin decreased insulin level in rats and mice with effects blocked by the melanocortin antagonist SHU9119[34,35]; (3) young lean MC4R knockout animals show hyperinsulinism before any confounding changes in body weight[34]; (4) humans with MC4R mutations have a relative hyperinsulinism compared with obese controls[36]; and (5) MC4Rs in brainstem parasympathetic neurones may be involved in the hyperinsulinemic response to obesity.

For MC4 receptors in brain stem parasympathetic neurones, using an elegant transgenic mouse model with global MC4R knockout combined with selective reexpression in targeted cell types, Rossi and colleagues showed that the hyperinsulinemia associated with loss of MC4 signaling was abrogated in mice reexpressing MC4R in Phox2b-expressing neurones. In contrast, MC4R reexpression in a wider repertoire of brain stem and intermediolateral column neurones (ChAT-expressing neurones) rescued broader glucose homeostatic responses (notably hepatic insulin sensitivity). These data suggest that melanocortinergic input into Phox2b expressing parasympathetic neurones in the brain stem controls insulin secretory responses in this model.[37]

CEPHALIC PHASE INSULIN RELEASE

The cephalic phase insulin response (sometimes referred to as the preabsorptive phase) refers to the rapid increase in insulin triggered by eating or anticipation of eating. Although it is a rapid and transient response (completing within 10 minutes) and is of low magnitude (perhaps 1%–2% of subsequent meal-induced insulin secretion), as detailed later, the cephalic phase insulin response may be of importance in determining the efficiency with which subsequent glucose disposal occurs.

Triggers may be olfactory, visual, gustatory, or oropharyngeal stimuli or indeed from higher centers from the anticipation of food.[38] They occur before any detectable increase in glucose in the blood stream so are a different mechanism from the studies described earlier examining hypothalamic control, in which a glucose load was delivered intravascularly. The concept that brain responds rapidly to the anticipation or arrival of food in the body to stimulate gastrointestinal responses is not new. At the start of the twentieth century, Pavlov showed increase in salivary, gastric, and pancreatic (exocrine) secretions in the oral cavity in dogs in anticipation of food or with arrival of food. In keeping with control from a brain gut circuit, vagotomy prevented gastric and pancreatic responses.[39,40] The cephalic phase of pancreatic secretion was then shown in humans for exocrine[41,42] and then later for insulin responses,[43] in part because of the greater challenges involved in the latter, requiring accurate insulin assays, rapid sampling methods, and appropriate control studies. In keeping with a nonnutrient-induced mechanism, cephalic phase insulin release can be stimulated by sham feeding or ingestion of nonmetabolizable food in rats.[44,45] Similarly in humans, sham feeding or nonmetabolizable sweeteners can stimulate cephalic phase insulin release.[43,46]

Underpinning the neural mechanism, cephalic phase insulin response is absent in the recently transplanted (and thus denervated) pancreas in rats[47] and humans,[48] but is present in decerebrate animals, in keeping with a brain stem circuitry activated by oral glucose.[49,50] Retrograde mapping studies from pancreas via the dorsal motor nucleus of the vagus showed sparse staining of the nucleus tractus solitarius, in keeping with gustatory afferents from the mouth activating a brain stem reflex.[9] Vagotomy[12,51,52] or atropine[53] diminish or abolish cephalic phase insulin responses, suggesting that the effects are predominantly vagal. Ahrens and Holst[54] found that ganglion blockade with trimethaphan had a greater inhibitory effect on early phase insulin release in healthy women than the cholinergic blocker, atropine, alone, suggesting that there may also be a significant noncholinergic mediation of the phenomenon.

How physiologically important is this rapid and small increase in insulin for glucose handling? The general importance of the early phase insulin release, whether triggered by brain or locally in the islets, was first suggested by a description of a negative correlation between the 30-minute insulin response to oral glucose and the 2-hour glucose value.[55] Brief administration of a small insulin dose during the first 15 minutes after food intake markedly improved glucose tolerance in patients with type 2 diabetes.[56] These and other similar observations did not distinguish between brain and local control of early phase insulin secretion. Examining specifically the contribution of cephalic phase insulin release required studies in which it was bypassed/blocked or mimicked. In studies in which oral intake was bypassed by intragastric[57] or intravenous routes,[58] oral stimulation aimed at triggering cephalic phase insulin release improved glucose handling. In support of these studies, using a pharmacologic approach to block cephalic phase insulin release either by ganglion blockade[54] or by infusing somatostatin[59] reduced the efficiency with which glucose was disposed of by the body, although clearly both of these agents have several potential actions. The mechanism by which a small and transient increase in circulating insulin can have an effect on subsequent glucose disposal after oral intake remains uncertain. Suggestions include an antilipolytic effect or the actions of intraportal insulin in inhibiting hepatic gluconeogenesis. Actions to prime target tissue insulin levels or stimulate mass glucose uptake seem less likely.

BRAIN CONTROL OF GLUCAGON RELEASE

At the simplest level, to help maintain circulating blood glucose levels, glucagon secretion increases as glucose levels decrease and decreases as glucose levels increase. The broader role of glucagon as part of the stress response is uncertain, although there is no doubt that glucagon levels increase in response to a variety of stressors, in which brain may play a role.[60] Most work examining control of glucagon has examined how secretion responds to changes in glucose, particularly hypoglycemia.

Multiple inputs help control glucagon release from α cells. Islets detect and respond rapidly to changes in ambient glucose, although it is unclear whether α cells directly sense changes in glucose. A significant body of evidence suggests that glucagon secretion is modulated by paracrine signaling from β and perhaps δ cells. Analogous to the incretin effect on insulin, GLP-1 acts to amplify suppression of glucagon by glucose arriving via the gastrointestinal tract.

However, in addition to these local factors, release of glucagon is controlled by autonomic factors originating in brain, either by direct sympathetic and parasympathetic innervation, as described earlier, or via changes in circulating catecholamines with preganglionic sympathetic neurones acting on chromaffin cells in the adrenal medulla via cholinergic nicotinic stimulation to increase release of catecholamines, principally circulating epinephrine, which stimulates glucagon release.[61]

The extent to which all of these possible influences on glucagon release interact and which factors (if any) predominate is uncertain. It seems likely that integrated control with both local and brain influences on islet secretion. For the autonomic factors during experimentally induced hypoglycemia (the best characterized physiologic/pathophysiologic situation with increased glucagon), studies suggest that there may be a redundancy, with each of the autonomic factors able to stimulate glucagon release independently. It is also possible that different influences may act at different levels of hypoglycemia. Local islet insulin switch-off occurs mostly in the low physiologic blood glucose range at glucose levels of more than 80 mg/dL. As glucose levels decrease less than this value, there is sequential activation of autonomic factors, initially parasympathetic and then sympathoadrenal (circulating catecholamine) stimulation, with sympathetic pancreatic activation occurring at the deepest levels of hypoglycemia less than 40 mg/dL.[61]

SITE OF HYPOGLYCEMIA SENSING

Selective catheterization studies in dogs allowing brain to be maintained at normoglycemic levels during systemic hypoglycemia found that this manipulation greatly attenuated counterregulatory responses, including glucagon.[62] This finding suggested that an important site of sensing a low glucose level and triggering glucagon release was located within the vascular supply of brain. Although further similar studies suggested that widespread brain regions may contribute to the control of glucagon response to hypoglycemia,[63] current thinking is that specialized glucose-sensing brain areas within the hypothalamus or brain stem[64] may play predominant roles. Hypoglycemia detection outside brain may also play a significant role in this process, perhaps via afferent information feeding in to key control centers.[65] It is also likely that stress modulation areas such as the amygdala and other brain limbic areas can modulate counterregulatory responses, including glucagon.[66,67] The current evidence for brain mechanisms underpinning the increase in glucagon release during hypoglycemia is described in more depth later.

A series of studies in the 1990s in rats suggested that hypothalamic brain areas, in particular the VMH, were of particular importance for triggering glucagon responses to hypoglycemia. Bilateral lesioning of the VMH by stereotaxic ibotenic acid injection abolished glucagon response to systemic hypoglycemia in rats.[68] Induction of local glucopenia by bilateral injections of 2-deoxyglucose into the VMH was able to trigger glucagon release.[69] Performing the opposite manipulation, local VMH glucose perfusion blocked glucagon response during systemic hypoglycemia in awake rats.[70] Consistent with these data, more recent work examining mice lacking vesicular transporters for glutamate neurotransmission in VMH SF1 neurones displayed defective glucagon response to hypoglycemia.[71]

MECHANISMS FOR SENSING HYPOGLYCEMIA AND TRIGGERING GLUCAGON RELEASE?

This section focuses on a model based on hypothalamic sensing of hypoglycemia with possible modulation by other sensors or stress-modulating areas within and outside brain. The main postulated mechanisms are outlined, again focusing on hypothalamic studies, although it is possible that similar glucose (hypoglycemia)-sensing apparatus operates in nonhypothalamic sensors. The efferent pathways to control α cells in pancreatic islets via brain stem autonomic outflow are described earlier. Later, the roles are discussed of adenosine triphosphate (ATP) gated potassium (K_{ATP}) channels and the inhibitory neurotransmitter γ-aminobutyric acid (GABA), GK, and BCl-associated death promoter (BAD), the low-affinity transporter GLUT2, the cellular energy sensor AMP-activated protein kinase (AMPK) and the neurotransmitter, GABA.

Several researchers have examined the potential parallels between pancreatic β-cell glucose sensing and the central (hypothalamic) mechanisms underpinning the detection of a decrease in blood glucose, specifically K_{ATP}, channels, GK, and GLUT2. K_{ATP} channels, a key part of the canonical glucose sensing in β cells, are widespread in brain and have been implicated in hypothalamic nutrient sensing. Infusion of sulfonylureas (to close K_{ATP} channels) into the hypothalamus attenuated glucagon response to hypoglycemia,[72] whereas brain delivery of K_{ATP} channel openers increased it.[73] Genetic inactivation of K_{ATP} channels in mice deficient for the Kir6.2 subunit of K_{ATP} channels showed reduced responses in glucose-sensing neurones in the VMH and defective glucagon (but not epinephrine) responses to both hypoglycemia and brain glucopenia. Isolated islets studied ex vivo showed similar glucagon responses to changes in glucose in knockout and wild-type mice, underpinning both the importance of K_{ATP} channels in brain for the generation of glucagon responses but also the role of brain hypoglycemia sensing in controlling how islet glucagon secretion responds to changes in glucose in the whole animal.[74] Changes in hypothalamic levels of GABA may also be important downstream mediators of changes in K_{ATP} channels to modulate centrally glucagon responses to hypoglycemia. Studies in which K_{ATP} channels in the VMH were opened or closed resulted in decreased or increase VMH GABA levels, respectively, corresponding in turn to amplification or suppression of glucagon and other counterregulatory responses to hypoglycemia.[75,76] In further studies from the same group,[77] microperfusion of glucose into the VMH of rats reduced decrease in VMH GABA and systemic glucagon and epinephrine responses to hypoglycemia. Effects of VMH glucose to suppress counterregulation were blocked by GABA A antagonist.

GK is also an important part of β-cell glucose detection. GK is found in brain, and agents acting on GK affect how glucose-sensing neurones respond in brain slice studies. In vivo, infusion of GK activators into VMH reduced glucagon response to hypoglycemia in rats.[78] In keeping with this finding, we recently presented data showing that I366F mice with a point mutation that reduces GK activity showed decreased glucagon responses to hypoglycemia.[79] In the β cell, the proapoptotic protein, BAD, acts via at least 2 different mechanisms (an interaction with GK and by its proapoptotic actions) to modulate insulin secretion. Acute genetic knockdown of BAD in brain impaired glucagon response to systemic glucoprivation in mice, although whether this is through altered GK effects remains unclear.[80]

The low-affinity glucose transporter GLUT2 is also believed to be an important part of the pancreatic β-cell glucose-sensing mechanism. GLUT2 has also been identified within brain. Using a transgenic model combining GLUT2 knockout with reexpression of GLUT1 within β cells (to restore insulin secretion), Thorens and colleagues[81] showed reduced glucagon responses to glucopenia associated with reduced activation in brain stem nuclei (dorsal vagal nucleus and nucleus tractus solitarius). In support of a brain role, glucagon responses were restored by central reexpression of GLUT2 but in glial rather than neuronal cells.[82]

The cellular energy sensor, AMPK, is found in brain, including glucose-responsive cells.[83] McCrimmon and colleagues[84] reported that genetic downregulation of AMPK in the VMH suppressed glucagon response to hypoglycemia in rats. These investigators also showed that pharmacologic activation of AMPK within the VMH by AICAR (5-aminoimidazole-4-carboxamide-1-β-D-ribofuranoside) boosted glucagon response to hypoglycemia in rats with impaired counterregulation.[85]

SUMMARY

Adequate levels of insulin and glucagon are critical for the maintenance of blood glucose homeostasis. In addition to the local mechanisms regulating islet secretion, accumulating evidence suggests pivotal roles for brain in directing the neural control of insulin and glucagon release. The precise nature of molecular mediators of the control of brain of islet secretion is being increasingly studied. The neuroanatomic networks involved in this pathway are also yet to be fully delineated.

A more detailed knowledge of the integrated control of islet function in the whole animal may pave the way for novel therapeutics to restore insulin and glucagon levels in glycemic disorders, particularly type 2 diabetes and impaired glucose counterregulation to hypoglycemia in types 1 and 2 diabetes.

REFERENCES

1. Kaneto A, Kosaka K, Nakao K. Effects of stimulation of the vagus nerve on insulin secretion. Endocrinology 1967;80(3):530–6.
2. Frohman LA, Ezdinli EZ, Javid R. Effect of vagotomy and vagal stimulation on insulin secretion. Diabetes 1967;16(7):443–8.
3. Bloom SR, Edwards AV. Pancreatic endocrine responses to stimulation via the sympathetic innervation. J Physiol 1975;245(2):120P–1P.
4. Pocai A, Lam TK, Gutierrez-Juarez R, et al. Hypothalamic K(ATP) channels control hepatic glucose production. Nature 2005;434(7036):1026–31.
5. Unger RH, Aquilar-Parado E, Muller WA, et al. Studies on pancreatic alpha cell function in normal and diabetic subjects. J Clin Invest 1970;49:837–48.
6. Lee Y, Wang MY, Du XQ, et al. Glucagon receptor knock-out prevents insulin-deficient type 1 diabetes in mice. Diabetes 2011;60:391–7.
7. Findlay JA, Gill JR, Lever JD, et al. Increased insulin output following stimulation of the vagal supply to the perfused rabbit pancreas. J Anat 1969;104(Pt 3):580.
8. Bloom SR, Edwards AV. The release of pancreatic glucagon and inhibition of insulin in response to stimulation of the sympathetic innervation. J Physiol 1975;253(1):157–73.
9. Streefland C, Maes FW, Bohus B. Autonomic brainstem projections to the pancreas: a retrograde transneuronal viral tracing study in the rat. J Auton Nerv Syst 1998;74:71–81.

10. Ahrén B, Taborsky GJ, Porte D. Neuropeptidergic versus cholinergic and adrenergic regulation of islet hormone secretion. Diabetologia 1986;29(12):827–36.
11. Ahren B, Paquette TL, Taborsky GJ Jr. Effect and mechanism of vagal nerve stimulation on somatostatin secretion in dogs. Am J Physiol 1986;250:E212–7.
12. Woods SC, Bernstein IL. Cephalic insulin response as a test for completeness of vagotomy to the pancreas. Physiol Behav 1980;24:485–8.
13. Karlsson S, Ahren B. Muscarinic receptor subtypes in carbachol-stimulated insulin and glucagon secretion in the mouse. J Auton Pharmacol 1993;13:439–46.
14. Gregersen S, Ahren B. Studies on the mechanisms by which gastrin releasing peptide stimulates insulin secretion from mouse islets. Pancreas 1996;12: 48–57.
15. Straub SG, Sharp GW. A wortmannin-sensitive signal transduction pathway is involved in the stimulation of insulin release by vasoactive intestinal polypeptide and pituitary adenylate cyclase-activating polypeptide. J Biol Chem 1996;271: 1660–8.
16. Bloom SR, Edwards AV. Characteristics of the neuroendocrine responses to stimulation of the splanchnic nerves in bursts in the conscious calf. J Physiol 1984; 346:533–45.
17. Skoglund G, Lundquist I, Ahren B. Selective alpha2-adrenoceptor activation by clonidine: effects on $^{45}Ca^{2+}$ efflux and insulin secretion from isolated rat islets. Acta Physiol Scand 1988;132:289–96.
18. Ahren B, Lundquist I. Effects of selective and nonselective beta-adrenergic agents on insulin secretion in vivo. Eur J Pharmacol 1981;71:93–104.
19. Ahren B. Autonomic regulation of islet hormone secretion. Implications for health and disease. Diabetologia 2000;43:393–410.
20. Jansen AS, Hoffman JL, Loewy AD. CNS sites involved in sympathetic and parasympathetic control of the pancreas: a viral tracing study. Brain Res 1997;766: 29–38.
21. Jansen AS, Nguyen XV, Karpitskiy V, et al. Central command neurons of the sympathetic nervous system: basis of the fight-or-flight response. Science 1995;270:644–6.
22. Strack AM, Sawyer WB, Platt KB, et al. CNS cell groups regulating the sympathetic outflow to adrenal gland as revealed by transneuronal cell body labeling with pseudorabies virus. Brain Res 1989;491:274–96.
23. Krowicki ZK, Hornby PJ. The nucleus raphe obscurus controls pancreatic hormone secretion in the rat. Am J Physiol 1995;268(6 Pt 1):E1128–34.
24. Krowicki ZK, Hornby PJ. Pancreatic polypeptide, microinjected into the dorsal vagal complex, potentiates glucose-stimulated insulin secretion in the rat. Regul Pept 1995;60(2–3):185–92.
25. Guillod-Maximin E, Lorsignol A, Alquier T, et al. Acute intracarotid glucose injection towards the brain induces specific c-fos activation in hypothalamic nuclei: involvement of astrocytes in cerebral glucose-sensing in rats. J Neuroendocrinol 2004; 16(5):464–71.
26. Leloup C, Magnan C, Benani A, et al. Mitochondrial reactive oxygen species are required for hypothalamic glucose sensing. Diabetes 2006;55(7):2084–90.
27. Clément L, Cruciani-Guglielmacci C, Magnan C, et al. Intracerebroventricular infusion of a triglyceride emulsion leads to both altered insulin secretion and hepatic glucose production in rats. Pflugers Arch 2002;445(3):375–80.
28. Cruciani-Guglielmacci C, Hervalet A, Douared L, et al. Beta oxidation in the brain is required for the effects of non-esterified fatty acids on glucose-induced insulin secretion in rats. Diabetologia 2004;47(11):2032–8.

29. Osundiji MA, Lam DD, Shaw J, et al. Brain glucose sensors play a significant role in the regulation of pancreatic glucose-stimulated insulin secretion. Diabetes 2012;61(2):321–8.
30. Rohner F, Dufour AC, Karakash C, et al. Immediate effect of lesion of the ventromedial hypothalamic area upon glucose-induced insulin secretion in anaesthetized rats. Diabetologia 1977;13(3):239–42.
31. Paranjape SA, Chan O, Zhu W, et al. Chronic reduction of insulin receptors in the ventromedial hypothalamus produces glucose intolerance and islet dysfunction in the absence of weight gain. Am J Physiol Endocrinol Metab 2011;301(5): E978–83.
32. Knauf C, Cani PD, Perrin C, et al. Brain glucagon-like peptide-1 increases insulin secretion and muscle insulin resistance to favor hepatic glycogen storage. J Clin Invest 2005;115(12):3554–63.
33. Calegari VC, Torsoni AS, Vanzela EC, et al. Inflammation of the hypothalamus leads to defective pancreatic islet function. J Biol Chem 2011;286(15):12870–80.
34. Fan W, Dinulescu DM, Butler AA, et al. The central melanocortin system can directly regulate serum insulin levels. Endocrinology 2000;141:3072–9.
35. Muzumdar R, Ma X, Yang X, et al. Physiologic effect of leptin on insulin secretion is mediated mainly through central mechanisms. FASEB J 2003;17(9):1130–2.
36. Martinelli CE, Keogh JM, Greenfield JR, et al. Obesity due to melanocortin 4 receptor (MC4R) deficiency is associated with increased linear growth and final height, fasting hyperinsulinemia, and incompletely suppressed growth hormone secretion. J Clin Endocrinol Metab 2011;96(1):E181–8.
37. Rossi J, Balthasar N, Olson D, et al. Melanocortin-4 receptors expressed by cholinergic neurons regulate energy balance and glucose homeostasis. Cell Metab 2011;13:195–204.
38. Goldfine ID, Abraira C, Gruenwald D, et al. Plasma insulin levels during imaginary food ingestion under hypnosis. Proc Soc Exp Biol Med 1970;133:274–86.
39. Pavlov I. The work of the digestive glands. London: Charles Griffin; 1902.
40. Wood J. The first Nobel prize for integrated systems physiology: Ivan Petrovich Pavlov, 1904. Physiology (Bethesda) 2004;19(6):326–30.
41. Defilippi CC, Solomon TE, Valenzuela JE. Pancreatic secretory response to sham feeding in humans. Digestion 1982;23(4):217–23.
42. Sarles H, Dani R, Prezelin G, et al. Cephalic phase of pancreatic secretion in man. Gut 1968;9(2):214–21.
43. Teff KL, Mattes RD, Engelman J, et al. Cephalic-phase insulin in obese and normal-weight men: relation to postprandial insulin. Metabolism 1993;42:1600–8.
44. Berthoud HR, Bereiter DA, Trimble ER, et al. Cephalic phase, reflex insulin secretion. Neuroanatomical and physiological characterization. Diabetologia 1981;20: 393–401.
45. Strubbe JH. Parasympathetic involvement in rapid meal-associated conditioned insulin secretion in the rat. Am J Physiol 1992;263:R615–8.
46. Bruce DG, Storlien LH, Furler SM, et al. Cephalic phase metabolic response in normal weight adults. Metabolism 1987;36:721–5.
47. Berthoud HR, Trimble ER, Siegel EG, et al. Cephalic-phase insulin secretion in normal and pancreatic islet-transplanted rats. Am J Physiol 1980;238:E336–40.
48. Secchi A, Caldara R, Caumo A, et al. Cephalic-phase insulin and glucagon release in normal subjects and in patients receiving pancreas transplantation. Metabolism 1995;44:1153–8.
49. Grill HJ, Berridge KC, Ganster DJ. Oral glucose is the prime elicitor of preabsorptive insulin secretion. Am J Physiol 1984;246:R88–95.

50. Flynn FW, Berridge KC, Grill HJ. Pre- and postabsorptive insulin secretion in chronic decerebrate rats. Am J Physiol 1986;250:R539–48.
51. Berthoud HR, Powley TL. Identification of vagal preganglionics that mediate cephalic phase insulin response. Am J Physiol 1990;258(2 Pt 2):R523–30.
52. Cox JE, Powley T. Prior vagotomy blocks VMH obesity in pair fed rats. Am J Physiol 1981;240:E573–83.
53. Berthoud HR, Jeanrenaud B. Sham feeding-induced cephalic phase insulin release in the rat. Am J Physiol 1982;242:E280–5.
54. Ahren B, Holst J. The cephalic insulin response to meal ingestion in humans is dependent on both cholinergic and noncholinergic mechanisms and is important for postprandial glycemia. Diabetes 2001;50:1030–8.
55. Mitrakou A, Kelley D, Mokam M, et al. Role of reduced suppression of glucose production and diminished early insulin release in impaired glucose tolerance. N Engl J Med 1992;326:22–9.
56. Bruttomesso D, Pianta A, Mari A, et al. Restoration of early rise in plasma insulin levels improves the glucose tolerance of type 2 diabetic patients. Diabetes 1999; 48:99–105.
57. Teff KL, Engelman K. Oral sensory stimulation improves glucose tolerance in humans: effects on insulin, C-peptide, and glucagon. Am J Physiol 1996;270: R1371–9.
58. Lorentzen M, Madsbad S, Kehlet H, et al. Effect of sham-feeding on glucose tolerance and insulin secretion. Acta Endocrinol (Copenh) 1987;115:84–6.
59. Calles-Escandon J, Robbins DC. Loss of early phase of insulin release in humans impairs glucose tolerance and blunts thermic effect of glucose. Diabetes 1987; 36:1167–72.
60. Jones BJ, Tan T, Bloom SR. Minireview: glucagon in energy and stress homoeostasis. Endocrinology 2012;153(3):1049–54.
61. Taborsky GJ Jr, Ahrén B, Havel PJ. Autonomic mediation of glucagon secretion during hypoglycemia: implications for impaired beta-cell responses in type 1 diabetes. Diabetes 1998;47:995–1005.
62. Biggers DW, Myers SR, Neal D, et al. Role of brain in counterregulation of insulin-induced hypoglycemia in dogs. Diabetes 1989;38(1):7–16.
63. Frizzell RT, Jones EM, Davis SN, et al. Counterregulation during hypoglycemia is directed by widespread brain regions. Diabetes 1993;42(9):1253–61.
64. Andrew SF, Dinh TT, Ritter S. Localized glucoprivation of hindbrain sites elicits corticosterone and glucagon secretion. Am J Physiol Regul Integr Comp Physiol 2007;292(5):R1792–849.
65. Saberi M, Bohland M, Donovan CM. Describe GS and GI. The locus for hypoglycemic detection shifts with the rate of fall in glycemia: the role of portal-superior mesenteric vein glucose sensing. Diabetes 2008;57(5):1380–6.
66. Zhou L, Podolsky N, Sang Z, et al. The medial amygdalar nucleus: a novel glucose-sensing region that modulates the counterregulatory response to hypoglycemia. Diabetes 2010;59(10):2646–52.
67. Hurst P, Garfield AS, Marrow C, et al. Recurrent hypoglycemia is associated with loss of activation in rat brain cingulate cortex. Endocrinology 2012;153(4): 1908–14.
68. Borg WP, During MJ, Sherwin RS, et al. Ventromedial hypothalamic lesions in rats suppress counterregulatory responses to hypoglycemia. J Clin Invest 1994;93(4): 1677–82.
69. Borg WP, Sherwin RS, During MJ, et al. Local ventromedial hypothalamus glucopenia triggers counterregulatory hormone release. Diabetes 1995;44(2):180–4.

70. Borg MA, Sherwin RS, Borg WP, et al. Local ventromedial hypothalamus glucose perfusion blocks counterregulation during systemic hypoglycemia in awake rats. J Clin Invest 1997;99(2):361–5.

71. Tong Q, Ye C, McCrimmon RJ, et al. Synaptic glutamate release by ventromedial hypothalamic neurons is part of the neurocircuitry that prevents hypoglycemia. Cell Metab 2007;5(5):383–93.

72. Evans ML, McCrimmon RJ, Flanagan DE, et al. Hypothalamic ATP-sensitive K^+ channels play a key role in sensing hypoglycemia and triggering counterregulatory epinephrine and glucagon responses. Diabetes 2004;53(10):2542–51.

73. McCrimmon RJ, Evans ML, Fan X, et al. Activation of ATP-sensitive K^+ channels in the ventromedial hypothalamus amplifies counterregulatory hormone responses to hypoglycemia in normal and recurrently hypoglycemic rats. Diabetes 2005;54(11):3169–74.

74. Miki T, Liss B, Minami K, et al. ATP-sensitive K^+ channels in the hypothalamus are essential for the maintenance of glucose homeostasis. Nat Neurosci 2001;4(5): 507–12.

75. Chan O, Lawson M, Zhu W, et al. ATP-sensitive $K(+)$ channels regulate the release of GABA in the ventromedial hypothalamus during hypoglycemia. Diabetes 2007;56:1120–6.

76. Chan O, Zhu W, Ding Y, et al. Sherwin RS blockade of GABA(A) receptors in the ventromedial hypothalamus further stimulates glucagon and sympathoadrenal but not the hypothalamo-pituitary-adrenal response to hypoglycemia. Diabetes 2006;55(4):1080–7.

77. Zhu W, Czyzyk D, Paranjape SA, et al. Glucose prevents the fall in ventromedial hypothalamic GABA that is required for full activation of glucose counterregulatory responses during hypoglycemia. Am J Physiol Endocrinol Metab 2010; 298(5):E971–7.

78. Levin BE, Becker TC, Eiki J-I, et al. Ventromedial hypothalamic glucokinase is an important mediator of the counterregulatory response to insulin-induced hypoglycemia. Diabetes 2008;57(5):1371–9.

79. Hurst PH, Marsh W, Riches CR, et al. Increased counter-regulatory responses to hypoglycaemia in mice with mutant glucokinase. Diabet Med 2011;28(Suppl 1):30–1; A84.

80. Osundiji MA, Godes ML, Evans ML, et al. BAD modulates counterregulatory responses to hypoglycemia and protective glucoprivic feeding. PLoS One 2011;6(12):e28016.

81. Thorens B, Guillam MT, Beermann F, et al. Transgenic reexpression of GLUT1 or GLUT2 in pancreatic beta cells rescues GLUT2-null mice from early death and restores normal glucose-stimulated insulin secretion. J Biol Chem 2000; 275(31):23751–8.

82. Marty N, Dallaporta M, Foretz M, et al. Regulation of glucagon secretion by glucose transporter type 2 (glut2) and astrocyte-dependent glucose sensors. J Clin Invest 2005;115(12):3545–53.

83. Beall C, Hamilton DL, Gallagher J, et al. Ashford ML mouse hypothalamic GT1-7 cells demonstrate AMPK-dependent intrinsic glucose-sensing behaviour. Diabetologia 2012;55(9):2432–44.

84. McCrimmon RJ, Shaw M, Fan X, et al. Key role for AMP-activated protein kinase in the ventromedial hypothalamus in regulating counterregulatory hormone responses to acute hypoglycemia. Diabetes 2008;57(2):444–50.

85. McCrimmon RJ, Fan X, Cheng H, et al. Activation of AMP-activated protein kinase within the ventromedial hypothalamus amplifies counterregulatory hormone responses in rats with defective counterregulation. Diabetes 2006;55(6):1755–60.

Defective Counterregulation and Hypoglycemia Unawareness in Diabetes

Mechanisms and Emerging Treatments

Candace M. Reno, PhD[a], Marina Litvin, MD[a], Amy L. Clark, DO[b], Simon J. Fisher, MD, PhD[a,c,*]

KEYWORDS

- Hypoglycemia • Unawareness • Glucose • Diabetes • Counterregulation • Brain
- Hypothalamus • Hypoglycemia-associated autonomic failure

KEY POINTS

- Hypoglycemia continues to be a major barrier to the achievement of long-term glucose control, causing recurrent morbidity in individuals with diabetes.
- Numerous sedulous research studies have begun to uncover the mechanisms by which the central nervous system responds and adapts to hypoglycemia.
- Understanding these mechanisms will undoubtedly lead to better management and therapies that reduce the risk for hypoglycemia, while still allowing patients to achieve the benefits associated with tight glycemic control.
- Given this pervasive barrier of hypoglycemia for the treatment of diabetes, physicians should discuss hypoglycemia prevention strategies with their patients, so they can have a better chance of achieving their goals of glucose control while avoiding the morbidity and mortality associated with hypoglycemia.

HYPOGLYCEMIA: THE CLINICAL PROBLEM

Poorly controlled diabetes is associated with vascular complications including renal failure, peripheral vascular disease, neuropathy, blindness, amputations, coronary artery disease, and stroke. Multiple large clinical trials have shown the benefits of intensifying glycemic control in preventing or delaying microvascular complications. These trials, however, consistently report significantly higher rates of hypoglycemia

[a] Division of Endocrinology, Metabolism & Lipid Research, Department of Medicine, Washington University, 660 South Euclid Avenue, St Louis, MO 63110, USA; [b] Division of Endocrinology and Diabetes, Department of Pediatrics, Washington University, 660 South Euclid Avenue, St Louis, MO 63110, USA; [c] Department of Cell Biology and Physiology, Washington University, 660 South Euclid Avenue, St Louis, MO 63110, USA
* Corresponding author. Division of Endocrinology, Metabolism & Lipid Research, Washington University in St Louis, Campus Box 8127, 660 South Euclid Avenue, St Louis, MO 63110.
E-mail address: sfisher@dom.wustl.edu

Endocrinol Metab Clin N Am 42 (2013) 15–38
http://dx.doi.org/10.1016/j.ecl.2012.11.005
0889-8529/13/$ – see front matter © 2013 Elsevier Inc. All rights reserved.

in patients who intensify their glycemic control.[1–5] Thus, hypoglycemia becomes the limiting factor for blood-glucose management in patients with diabetes, and precludes the attainment of microvascular benefits associated with tight glycemic control.

INCIDENCE OF HYPOGLYCEMIA

Compared with earlier self-reported and glucometer-based studies, studies based on continuous glucose monitoring more accurately assess the true incidence of hypoglycemia. In reasonably well-controlled patients with type 1 diabetes (HbA1c 7.6%), biochemical hypoglycemia (<60 mg/dL) averaged a disconcertingly high 2.1 times per 24 hours.[6] Of note, even in the group of people who reported intact hypoglycemia awareness, biochemically confirmed hypoglycemia failed to elicit symptoms 62% of the time.[6] Thus, symptomatic hypoglycemia underestimates the true incidence of hypoglycemia, and hypoglycemia awareness is not an "all or none" phenomenon.

As discussed in this article, episodes of moderate hypoglycemia are not without clinical consequences. Recurrent episodes of moderate hypoglycemia can lead to decreased sympathoadrenal responses and decreased awareness of hypoglycemia, collectively termed hypoglycemia-associated autonomic failure (HAAF),[7] which leads to an increased risk of more frequent and more severe episodes of hypoglycemia.

SEVERE HYPOGLYCEMIA

Severe hypoglycemia is defined clinically as occurring when the patient requires assistance from another individual to correct hypoglycemia. For insulin-treated diabetic patients, severe hypoglycemia has a high prevalence (46% and 25%) and high incidence (3.2 and 0.7 episodes per person-year) for people with type 1 and type 2 diabetes, respectively.[8] Severe hypoglycemia is associated with excess morbidity and mortality[7]; it can alter brain structure[9] and cause brain damage,[10,11] cognitive dysfunction,[12,13] and even sudden death.[14] It is estimated that between 6% and 10% of patients with type 1 diabetes die from hypoglycemia.[15–17] The mechanism by which low glucose levels lead to sudden death has not been entirely worked out, but seems to be related to intensive sympathetic activation leading to fatal cardiac arrhythmias.[18,19]

THE COUNTERREGULATORY RESPONSE TO HYPOGLYCEMIA

Because the brain is continuously dependent on peripheral glucose for metabolism, robust counterregulatory mechanisms exist to rapidly increase blood-glucose levels to protect the body from the pathologic consequences of hypoglycemia. In the setting of absolute or relative hyperinsulinemia, the counterregulatory response (CRR) is normally initiated when glucose levels fall below 80 mg/dL. The CRR to hypoglycemia normally includes suppression of endogenous insulin secretion and increase the secretion of glucagon, catecholamines (epinephrine, norepinephrine), cortisol, and growth hormone, which together act to increase plasma glucose levels by stimulating hepatic glucose production and limiting the use of glucose in peripheral tissues (**Fig. 1**).

GLUCAGON RESPONSE TO HYPOGLYCEMIA

Normally as blood-glucose levels decrease, increased glucagon secretion from the pancreatic α cells and decreased insulin secretion are the primary counterregulatory mechanisms by which hepatic glucose production is increased. Insulin-deficient diabetes results in an acquired defect of the glucagon response.[20] Several mechanisms have been proposed to explain this phenomenon, including defective

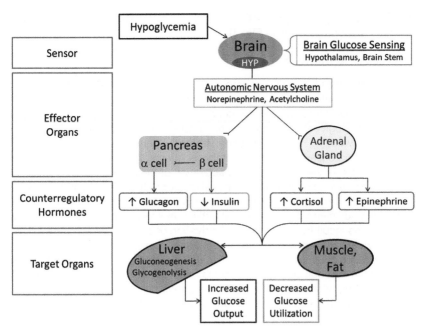

Fig. 1. The counterregulatory response to hypoglycemia. Hypoglycemia is first sensed in various brain regions including the hypothalamus and brainstem. Low glucose in these brain regions stimulates the autonomic nervous system to release norepinephrine and acetylcholine at postganglionic nerve terminals and induce symptoms of hypoglycemia (hypoglycemia awareness). A principal counterregulatory response is the secretion of glucagon, which may be stimulated by various mechanisms including independent α-cell glucose sensing, autonomic innervation, epinephrine stimulation, and a reduction of intra-islet insulin secretion. Via autonomic stimulation, epinephrine is released from the adrenal medulla. Not shown is the hypothalamic-pituitary-adrenal axis by which the release of corticotropin from the pituitary stimulates cortisol release from the adrenal cortex. The cumulative effect of the sympathetic nervous system and counterregulatory hormones at the level of the liver is to increase hepatic gluconeogenesis and glycogenolysis, whereas the effect at muscle and adipose tissue is to decrease peripheral glucose use.

α-cell glucose sensing, absent decrements in insulin secretion (intra-islet crosstalk), and reduced autonomic stimulation (recently reviewed in Refs.[21,22]). Elevated intra-islet somatostatin within the diabetic pancreas may also play a role in limiting the glucagon response to hypoglycemia, because pharmacologic antagonism of the somatostatin receptor can restore the glucagon response to hypoglycemia in diabetic rats.[23]

SYMPATHETIC AND ADRENAL MEDULLARY COUNTERREGULATORY RESPONSE

In response to hypoglycemia, patients with type 1 diabetes and advanced type 2 diabetes are not able to suppress circulating (exogenous) insulin levels or increase glucagon secretion.[20] Thus, patients with diabetes rely extensively on the sympathoadrenal system as their primary counterregulatory defense against hypoglycemia.[19] Adrenergic activation leads to the release of norepinephrine at nerve terminals located throughout the periphery. Adrenergic stimulation of the adrenal glands stimulates epinephrine release. Activation of the adrenergic system combats falling glucose levels by increasing glucose production, reducing peripheral glucose use, and eliciting symptoms of hypoglycemia (see **Fig. 1**).

HYPOGLYCEMIA AWARENESS

Exigent hypoglycemia is usually accompanied by characteristic signs and symptoms, which prompt the patient to take corrective action. Neurogenic symptoms occur as a result of activation of the autonomic nervous system by hypoglycemia, and lead to perception of hypoglycemia (hypoglycemia awareness) by the patient. These symptoms include sweating, hunger, tingling, tremors, palpitations, nervousness, and anxiety. As characterized in adrenalectomized patients, these neurogenic symptoms of hypoglycemia are chiefly the result of activation of the sympathetic neural system, rather than epinephrine or norepinephrine release from the adrenal gland.[24] Thus the unawareness of hypoglycemic symptoms in patients with diabetes is inexorably linked to exiguous sympathetic neuronal activation. On the other hand, neuroglycopenic symptoms result from the brain's deprivation of glucose, and may be exhibited as warmth, weakness, altered mental status, drowsiness, seizures, or even coma or death.[25] Autonomic symptoms of hypoglycemia tend to occur at higher thresholds (58 mg/dL) than neuroglycopenic symptoms, which tend to occur at 51 mg/dL.[26] In the setting of progressive hypoglycemia, awareness of autonomic symptoms generally occurs before the development of profound neuroglycopenic symptoms, allowing the patient a window of opportunity to initiate corrective action to ameliorate hypoglycemia before global cognitive impairments limit behavioral responses and hypoglycemia becomes life threatening.

ANATOMY OF BRAIN GLUCOSE SENSING

Although all brain cells use glucose, only a few specialized neurons in the brain truly sense and respond to reduced glucose supply. Rodent studies indicate that glucose is sensed in brain regions known to be important in metabolism and energy homeostasis, particularly in the hypothalamus, where glucose-sensing neurons are located.[27,28] Most studies to date indicate that it is the hypothalamus that principally initiates (or at least coordinates) the CRR to stimulate hormone secretion in the pituitary gland, pancreas, and adrenal glands, resulting in a coordinated response. Clinical studies confirm the importance of the hypothalamus as a critical glucose-sensing area because blood flow to the hypothalamus increases significantly during hypoglycemia, even before the levels of counterregulatory hormones increase.[29] Within the hypothalamus, key regions that respond to changes in circulating glucose levels are the ventromedial hypothalamus (VMH), which contains the ventromedial nucleus (VMN) and the arcuate nucleus (ARC).[30] Studies show that glucose infusion into the VMH in the setting of peripheral hypoglycemia blunts the epinephrine response to hypoglycemia.[31,32] These studies indicate that decreases in glucose are detected by the VMH and are required to fully activate the sympathoadrenal response to hypoglycemia (**Fig. 2**).

The VMH contains glucose-excitatory (GE, which increase neuronal activity in response to glucose) and glucose-inhibited (GI, which decrease neuronal activity in response to glucose) neurons.[33] Similarities and differences between GI and GE neurons with regard to glucose metabolic and electrophysiologic properties have been reviewed.[34] It is thought that in response to hypoglycemia, concerted activation of GI neurons and suppression of GE neurons, as an initiating part of a neural network, results in a coordinated efferent process that activates the sympathoadrenal response (**Fig. 3**).

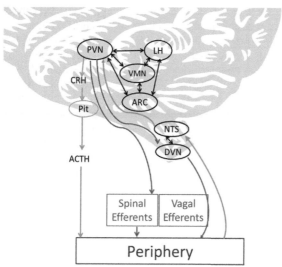

Fig. 2. Afferent glucose-sensing pathways, neural integration, and efferent autonomic pathways that mediate the counterregulatory response to hypoglycemia. During hypoglycemia, the initiation and coordination of the counterregulatory response is mediated by a network of glucose-sensing neurons in the hypothalamus, including the ventromedial nucleus (VMN), arcuate nucleus (ARC), and lateral hypothalamus (LH). Glucose sensing also occurs in the nucleus tractus solitarius (NTS) and dorsal motor nucleus of the vagus (DVN) in the hindbrain. The NTS also receives afferent information from peripheral glucose sensors, including the portal vein. Hypothalamic and hindbrain neural networks project to the paraventricular nucleus of the hypothalamus (PVN) to elicit autonomic and neuroendocrine counterregulatory responses. Although not directly glucose sensing, parvicellular neurons in the PVN initiate sympathetic autonomic responses via preganglionic spinal efferents. Parasympathetic (vagal) innervation is relayed from the PVN to the DVN, which then relays to peripheral organs. In addition, the hypothalamic-pituitary-adrenal axis is also initiated from a distinct set of medial parvicellular neurons within the PVN that secretes corticotropin-releasing hormone (CRH). CRH acts on the anterior pituitary (Pit) to stimulate the secretion of adrenocorticotropic hormone (ACTH), which circulates to the adrenal cortex to increase cortisol secretion. Interneurons involved in the neural glucose sensing and autonomic response network are shown in black. Afferent glucose-sensing pathways are shown in green. Efferent autonomic responses to hypoglycemia are shown in brown. The postganglionic vagal parasympathetic efferent pathway is shown in red. The hypothalamic-pituitary-adrenal axis is shown in blue.

Other glucose-sensing neurons have been discovered in regions outside the hypothalamus. Within the brainstem, the nucleus tractus solitarius (NTS), the area postrema (AP), the dorsal motor nucleus of the vagus (DVN), and the subfornical region have been shown to contain glucose-sensing neurons.[35–37] Other peripheral glucose-sensing neurons (ie, within the portal/mesenteric vein, gut, and carotid bodies) ascend via afferent neurons to the brainstem (NTS), which projects anteriorly to the paraventricular nucleus (PVN) of the hypothalamus (see **Fig. 2**).[30]

Activation of the PVN seems to be critically important for activating several aspects of the stress CRRs, including (1) release of corticotropin-releasing hormone, which acts on the anterior pituitary to release corticotropin, (2) innervation of the DVN to regulate the vagal parasympathetic efferent neurons, and perhaps most importantly, (3) direct activation of sympathetic nerves in the spinal cord (see **Fig. 2**). Failure to

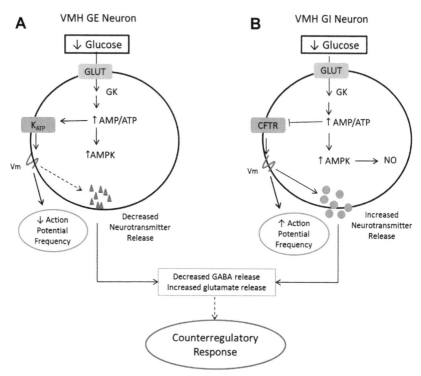

Fig. 3. Glucose-sensing neurons of the ventromedial hypothalamus (VMH). (*A*) VMH glucose-excited (GE) neurons are activated in response to increasing glucose. In a setting of low glucose, decreased glucose entry into the GE neuron through glucose transporters (GLUT) leads to decreased phosphorylation by glucokinase (GK), leading to an increase in the adenosine monophosphate/adenosine triphosphate (AMP/ATP) ratio, thus increasing the activity of AMP-activated protein kinase (AMPK) and stimulating K_{ATP} channel activation. Activation of K_{ATP} channels leads to decreased membrane depolarization and decreased action-potential frequency and neurotransmitter release, in particular γ-amino-butyric acid (GABA), thus leading to activation of the hypoglycemic counterregulatory response. (*B*) VMH glucose-inhibited (GI) neurons are activated in response to decreasing glucose. Decreased glucose entry into neurons leads to an increase in the AMP/ATP ratio and activation of AMPK, activating the formation of nitric oxide (NO), which can act as a neurotransmitter. Increased AMP/ATP also inhibits a chloride channel, thought to be the cystic fibrosis transmembrane conductance regulator (CFTR), leading to membrane depolarization, increased action-potential frequency, and neurotransmitter release, including glutamate, which leads to activation of the counterregulatory response. GABA and glutamate can potentially be secreted from both GE and GI neurons on their activation, but a decrease in GABA levels is required for full activation of the counterregulatory response.

activate PVN neurons is a common finding in animal models that exhibit impaired CRRs to hypoglycemia.[38,39]

CELLULAR BIOLOGY OF BRAIN GLUCOSE SENSING

The brain contains different isoforms of glucose transporters responsible for neuronal and astrocyte glucose uptake. The ubiquitous GLUT1 and the neural-specific GLUT3 are the primary isoforms present in the brain that are responsible for glucose transport across the blood-brain barrier and into the brain. Based on discrete regional expression, the potential contribution of other glucose transporters has been investigated. A role for GLUT2 in mediating glucose sensing in the central nervous system (CNS) has been proposed.[40] Also, a role for insulin-sensitive GLUT4 in mediating brain glucose sensing and the CRR to hypoglycemia was evident in recent reports from the authors' laboratory showing that in response to hypoglycemia, brain GLUT4 knockout mice have (1) impaired epinephrine and glucagon responses, (2) impaired neuronal activation within the hypothalamus, and (3) impaired glucose sensing in GI neurons.[41] Further research is needed to help understand how differential regional expression of the various glucose transporters regulates the CRR to hypoglycemia.

Once glucose enters the cells it is phosphorylated by glucokinase, an enzyme that has been shown to play an important role in mediating hypothalamic glucose sensing.[42,43] Metabolism of glucose increases the intracellular adenosine triphosphate (ATP) to adenosine monophosphate (AMP) ratio, which in turn regulates the activity of a key metabolic sensor, AMP-activated protein kinase (AMPK). During acute hypoglycemia, increased AMPK activity is hypothesized to lead to chloride ion (cystic fibrosis transmembrane conductance regulator, CFTR) channel closure, neuronal depolarization, and neurotransmitter release in GI neurons (see **Fig. 3**).[44,45] However, in GE neurons, downstream of glucose metabolism, it is the activation of K_{ATP} channels that increases the sympathoadrenal response to hypoglycemia.[33,34,46] Thus, pharmacologic or genetic disruption of the metabolic[41,42,44] or electrophysiologic[33,34,45] properties in these critical VMH glucose-sensing neurons can lead to impaired hypoglycemic counterregulation.

HORMONAL AND NEUROHORMONAL REGULATION OF CNS GLUCOSE SENSING

The intrinsic glucose-sensing/metabolism properties of glucose-sensing neurons in the VMH can be acutely modified by the action of circulating hormones. Both leptin and insulin cross the blood-brain barrier and have been shown to acutely activate K_{ATP} channels in glucose-sensing hypothalamic neurons.[47] In the setting of hypoglycemia, insulin has been shown to act in the brain to augment the CRR.[48] Furthermore, neuronal insulin receptor knockout (NIRKO) mice have impaired hypoglycemic counterregulation, characterized by a blunted epinephrine and norepinephrine response.[39] Consistent with insulin exerting its effect primarily in the hypothalamus, NIRKO mice have impaired glucose sensing in VMH GI neurons and impaired activation of PVN neurons in response to hypoglycemia.[39] Together, these studies demonstrate that central insulin signaling plays an important role in regulating the normal CRR to hypoglycemia. Other, slower-acting hormones, including nuclear receptor transcription activators such as cortisol (discussed later), may also exert more long-term effects in regulating hypothalamic glucose sensing.

As the blood-glucose level decreases, glucose levels within the brain also decrease. A decrease in glucose levels within the VMH is associated with increased norepinephrine release in the VMH and the initiation of the CRR to hypoglycemia.[49,50] Adrenergic receptors within the brain, particularly the VMH, are important mediators that trigger the sympathoadrenal response to hypoglycemia.[51] It is likely that increased or decreased catecholaminergic neurotransmitter output from other glucose-sensing neurons (perhaps portal-mesenteric glucose-sensitive afferents[52]) are integrated in the VMH to either amplify or suppress, respectively, the sympathoadrenal response to hypoglycemia.

DEFECTIVE COUNTERREGULATION AND HYPOGLYCEMIA UNAWARENESS IN PEOPLE WITH DIABETES AND RECURRENT HYPOGLYCEMIA

As noted earlier, in people with type 1 and advanced type 2 diabetes, impaired hypoglycemic counterregulation is noted by a failure to both suppress circulating insulin and increase glucagon secretion, which leads to an increased reliance on the sympathoadrenal response as the primary CRR.[53,54] Recurrent hypoglycemia further impairs the sympathoadrenal response as part of a vicious cycle, making diabetic patients vulnerable to more severe episodes of hypoglycemia.[7,20] In addition, recurrent hypoglycemia induces impairments in brain glucose sensing on a cellular basis in glucose-sensing VMH neurons[55] as well as on a whole-body basis, noted clinically by both impaired sympathoadrenal responsiveness and hypoglycemia unawareness (**Fig. 4**). Hypoglycemia unawareness increases the incidence of severe hypoglycemia 6-fold for type 1 diabetic patients[56] and 17-fold for type 2 diabetic patients.[57] Although approximately 20% of type 1 diabetic patients report hypoglycemia unawareness,[56] this value is most certainly an underestimation, as even diabetic patients who have intact hypoglycemia awareness are often unaware of biochemically confirmed hypoglycemia.[6]

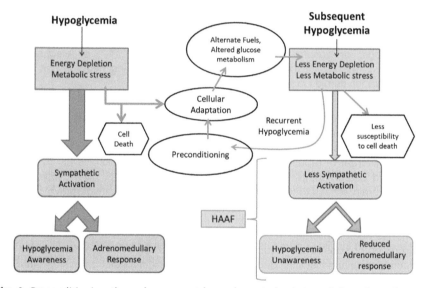

Fig. 4. Preconditioning through recurrent hypoglycemia leads to cellular adaptation and hypoglycemia-associated autonomic failure (HAAF). Hypoglycemia is a state of energy depletion that leads to metabolic stress. Sympathetic activation leads to symptoms of hypoglycemia awareness and the adrenomedullary response. The normal response to hypoglycemia is a cellular adaptation, assuming the energy depletion and metabolic stress was not enough to induce cell death. The mechanism by which cellular adaptation occurs is unclear, but may include the use of alternative fuels (such as lactate) and/or an enhanced glucose transport/phosphorylation/metabolism. During a subsequent hypoglycemic episode, the adapted cell experiences less marked energy depletion and less metabolic stress, thus making the cells less susceptible to death. Less intracellular energy depletion leads to impaired sympathetic activation, resulting in hypoglycemia unawareness and a reduced adrenomedullary response to subsequent hypoglycemia, collectively known as HAAF. Preconditioning through recurrent hypoglycemia, paradoxically, acts to render an individual more prone to, but less vulnerable to, an episode of severe hypoglycemia.

The mechanisms by which recurrent hypoglycemia leads to altered CNS glucose sensing, impaired sympathoadrenal activation, and hypoglycemia unawareness remain an active area of investigation.[58] Several potential mediators being investigated include (1) actions of hormones released during hypoglycemia (cortisol, epinephrine, opioids), (2) cell autonomous changes in substrate metabolism, and (3) altered neuronal circuitry/neurotransmitter release. These mechanisms are not mutually exclusive. Better understanding of these mechanisms will aid in developing therapeutic strategies to prevent hypoglycemia unawareness in insulin-treated patients with diabetes.

PERIPHERAL MEDIATORS OF HAAF AND HYPOGLYCEMIA UNAWARENESS
Cortisol

The hypothalamic-pituitary-adrenal axis involves a family of neuropeptides that regulate glucocorticoid (cortisol) secretion during stress. Corticotropin-releasing hormone agonists have been shown to impair the CRR to subsequent hypoglycemia, suggesting a possible mechanistic role in mediating HAAF.[59] The hypoglycemia-associated increase in systemic corticosteroids has been proposed to feedback to the hypothalamus and thereby to potentially contribute to HAAF.[60–62] It remains controversial as to whether the endogenous hypercortisolemia associated with the CRR is of sufficient magnitude to blunt the CRR to hypoglycemia.[63,64]

Catecholamines

It has been well established that antecedent hypoglycemia induces a blunted epinephrine response to a subsequent episode of hypoglycemia. A study by Ramanathan and Cryer[65] showed that intravenous infusion of adrenergic blockers (phentolamine and propranolol) on day 1 of hypoglycemia prevented the induction of counterregulatory failure in the subsequent response on day 2 of hypoglycemia. This study implies that HAAF is induced by antecedent sympathoadrenal responses to hypoglycemia, and possibly the antecedent sympathoadrenal response to exercise, as discussed later. Extending these findings to their potential pharmacologic and therapeutic implications, an apparent dichotomy emerges whereby blocking the action of catecholamines (presumably within the CNS) may protect against subsequent hypoglycemic bouts by limiting the development of HAAF; unfortunately, however, blocking the action of catecholamines in the periphery would tend to increase the severity of acute hypoglycemia. Perhaps future pharmacologic treatment of recurrent severe hypoglycemia will involve the development of selective adrenergic receptor modulators that favorably alter CNS-mediated CRRs without adversely altering the beneficial peripheral effects of the sympathoadrenal response.

Opioids

Opioid signaling in the CNS has also been implicated in the development of impaired sympathoadrenal responses in people with type 1 diabetes. Naloxone, an opioid receptor blocker, augmented the sympathoadrenal response to hypoglycemia[66] and, when infused during antecedent hypoglycemia, it prevented the development of the hypoglycemia-associated reduced epinephrine response.[67] Mechanistically, naloxone may preserve the CRR to hypoglycemia by reprogramming metabolic genes to use alternative fuels instead of glucose.[68] Together, these preclinical and clinical studies implicate that the increase in endogenous opioids that occurs during hypoglycemia have a pathologic role in mediating the adrenomedullary defect associated with HAAF, and a potential therapeutic role for opioid receptor blockade to protect against HAAF.

Exercise

The inability to decrease circulating insulin during exercise puts people with type 1 diabetes at increased risk for hypoglycemia during or after exercise. Furthermore, antecedent exercise can decrease sympathoadrenal responses to subsequent hypoglycemia.[69] It is interesting that despite this reduced epinephrine response to hypoglycemia following exercise, symptoms of hypoglycemia are not reduced, suggesting that there can be a distinction between hypoglycemia awareness and the counterregulatory adrenal response. In addition, during stress, including hypoglycemia and exercise, the opioid β-endorphin is released to activate the sympathoadrenal response. In a recent study, healthy volunteers who exercised and had elevated endorphin levels had impaired epinephrine and norepinephrine responses during hypoglycemia the following day.[70] Thus, the impaired adrenomedullary response to hypoglycemia induced by antecedent hypoglycemia or exercise may be mediated by endogenous opioid action within the CNS. From a therapeutic perspective, therefore, blocking the actions of endogenous opioids may protect against exercise-induced autonomic failure.

Sleep

Nocturnal hypoglycemia is very common in patients with type 1 diabetes. It has a prevalence rate of up to 68%[71] and has an incidence of once every third night.[72] While sleeping, subjects with type 1 diabetes have a significantly reduced epinephrine response to hypoglycemia[73] and reduced awakening from sleep during hypoglycemia, in comparison with nondiabetics.[74] Thus the state of sleep induces a transient, additional, HAAF-like syndrome, characterized by hypoglycemia unawareness and an impaired adrenomedullary response to hypoglycemia.

If a diabetic patient is unable to wake up and take corrective actions, nocturnal hypoglycemia can be potentially life threatening. Tattersall and Gill[75] have reported the unexplained overnight deaths of otherwise healthy young people with type 1 diabetes, often referred to as the "dead-in-bed syndrome." Recently, the overnight death of a young man with type 1 diabetes confirmed, via retrospective continuous glucose monitoring, that the dead-in-bed syndrome is associated with severe hypoglycemia.[14,75]

ALTERNATIVE SUBSTRATE METABOLISM
Glycogen Supercompensation

It has been hypothesized that increased glycogen stores in astrocytes might contribute to hypoglycemia unawareness and impaired sympathoadrenal responses by supplementing glucosyl units for CNS metabolism during periods of systemic hypoglycemia. Studies in rats and humans have shown that brain glycogen content is increased following one or more episodes of hypoglycemia[76,77] or 2-deoxyglucose–induced neuroglycopenia.[78] At present, much controversy exists in this field because subsequent studies have shown that glycogen content in the rat brain is not elevated after acute or recurrent hypoglycemia[79] and that lower, not higher, glycogen levels exist in diabetic patients.[80] It is hoped that improved techniques in measuring the turnover of brain glycogen in vivo both during and after hypoglycemia will resolve these apparent discrepant results. The more important question to be addressed is whether changes to levels of brain glycogen (induced via physiologic or pharmacologic means) will offer people who suffer from recurrent hypoglycemia a beneficial therapeutic advantage in preserving both sympathoadrenal responses and hypoglycemia awareness.

Enhanced Glucose Metabolism

Alterations in glucose transport or glucose metabolism as a result of repeated exposure to hypoglycemia have been postulated to be a potential mediator of HAAF. Increased glucose transport to sustain metabolic demands during hypoglycemia is supported by studies in rats that show increased expression of glucose transporters in the brain after acute hypoglycemia[81] and after recurrent hypoglycemia.[82] The next important metabolic regulator in glucose-sensing neurons is the enzyme glucokinase, the expression level of which is also upregulated in the setting of recurrent hypoglycemia.[42] Consistent with an upregulation of glucose transport or glucokinase activity, recurrent hypoglycemia has been shown to increase hypothalamic glucose phosphorylation.[83] Therefore, repeated exposure to hypoglycemia may upregulate the capacity for glucose metabolism (including increased glucose transporters, glucokinase activity, and glucose phosphorylation) during subsequent hypoglycemia. This process simultaneously limits neuroglycopenia and induces hypoglycemia unawareness at the cellular level in glucose-sensing neurons, ultimately resulting in a diminished sympathoadrenal response.

Although it is supported in some[42,82,83] but not all[84] rodent models, altered glucose transport/metabolism as a cause for hypoglycemia unawareness is less well substantiated in humans. During hypoglycemia, type 1 diabetic patients had similar glucose metabolism in the brain in comparison with healthy controls.[85] Patients with hypoglycemia unawareness seem to have normal global brain glucose metabolism, although several studies have identified specific brain regions that exhibit decreased glucose uptake, including the subthalamic brain region involving the hypothalamus,[86] the prefrontal cortex,[87] the amygdala, and orbitofrontal cortex.[88] Iatrogenic hypoglycemia that induces HAAF also did not increase global brain glucose transport in healthy patients,[89] but was associated with significantly greater synaptic activity in the dorsal midline thalamus.[90] Further clinical studies using enhanced positron emission tomography and magnetic resonance imaging technologies to examine regional brain glucose uptake/metabolism in patients with type 1 diabetes with and without HAAF will help define the brain regions pathologically linked to this clinical syndrome.

Alternative Fuel Hypothesis

In the setting of reduced glucose supply from the periphery, the brain may be able to decrease its reliance on circulating glucose and maintain its metabolic processes by increasing its uptake of alternative carbon fuels, such as ketones or lactate.[91] Lactate from astrocytes can be taken up into neurons via monocarboxylate transporters (MCT), and is hypothesized to support oxidative phosphorylation during times of glucose deficit.[84,91,92] During a hypoglycemic clamp, type 1 diabetic patients had 2-fold higher brain lactate concentrations than control subjects, indicating increased uptake of lactate in the brain.[93] If, in response to recurrent hypoglycemia, the brain has adapted in such a way as to meet its metabolic demands by using relatively more lactate rather than circulating glucose, the neurons' sufficed metabolic demands likely blunt its ability to sense and respond to subsequent hypoglycemia, resulting in impaired sympathetic activation and hypoglycemia unawareness (see **Fig. 4**).

Altered Neuronal Communication

γ-Aminobutyric acid (GABA) is a potent inhibitory neurotransmitter. Hypothalamic GABA levels normally decrease during hypoglycemia,[94] thereby relinquishing a tonic inhibitory effect on VMH neurons and allowing the generation of the CRR. Both diabetic rats and recurrently hypoglycemic rats have higher basal levels of VMH GABA that fail to decrease normally during subsequent hypoglycemia, which correlates with the reduced glucagon and epinephrine responses.[95,96] These results indicate that altered GABA tone may be an important common mediator in the development of HAAF, especially in diabetic patients, and drugs that selectively target GABA secretion or receptor binding may improve sympathoadrenal responses to hypoglycemia.

ADAPTATIONS TO RECURRENT HYPOGLYCEMIA: ADAPTIVE OR MALADAPTIVE?

Repetitive hypoglycemia induces a state of hypoglycemic tolerance whereby lower and lower levels of blood glucose are needed to elicit symptomatic responses and CRRs. From a teleologic perspective, brain adaptations that occur in response to repetitive hypoglycemia endeavor to maintain neuronal/cognitive function via sufficing CNS metabolic needs in the setting of another episode of hypoglycemia. Unfortunately, these adaptations ultimately reduce neuronal efferent signals, thereby limiting sympathoadrenal responses, and induce a state of hypoglycemia unaware-ness.[7] Metabolic adaptations in patients with hypoglycemia unawareness allow cognitive function at dangerously low blood-sugar levels, but do so at the perilous risk of a precipitous neuroglycopenic coma. By reducing awareness and counterregu-lation to subsequent hypoglycemia, HAAF jeopardizes patient safety and should therefore be considered a maladaptive response.[7,97] However, hypoglycemic toler-ance induced by recurrent hypoglycemia may induce some unexpected beneficial adaptations. The authors' group has shown that adaptations associated with recur-rent antecedent hypoglycemia protect the brain against severe hypoglycemia-induced brain damage and cognitive decline.[11] Thus, similar to the phenomenon of preconditioning, recurrent bouts of moderate hypoglycemia might, paradoxically, render an individual more prone to, but less vulnerable to, an episode of severe hypo-glycemia. If a neuroprotective effect of hypoglycemic preconditioning were to be extrapolated to the clinical setting, it may explain the seemingly incongruous clinical findings that intensively treated patients, who experience recurrent hypoglycemia, may be paradoxically protected from severe hypoglycemia–induced brain damage and cognitive dysfunction.[16] Of course recurrent hypoglycemia should not be advo-cated clinically, but defining the mechanisms of how recurrent hypoglycemia leads to beneficial adaptations could lead to the development of pharmacologic agents that will help protect against the morbidity and mortality associated with severe hypoglycemia.[11,98]

PREVENTION OF HYPOGLYCEMIA, DEFECTIVE COUNTERREGULATION, AND HYPOGLYCEMIA UNAWARENESS

Identification of patients with risk factors for severe hypoglycemia is a critical step in the prevention of hypoglycemia. Type 1 diabetic patients with hypoglycemia unaware-ness and impaired counterregulation are more likely to be older, have diabetes of longer duration, and have lower HbA1c.[99,100] Gender may also contribute to risk for hypoglycemia. The blunted CRR to hypoglycemia in women,[101] likely mediated by estrogen,[102] uniquely increases the risk for hypoglycemia in women.[103]

Strategies for the prevention of hypoglycemia include frequent self-monitoring of blood-glucose levels and patient education regarding insulin analogues, dose adjust-ments for anticipated exercise and carbohydrate consumption, and the use of tech-nology for insulin administration and blood-glucose monitoring (ie, insulin pumps and continuous glucose sensors).

AVOIDANCE OF HYPOGLYCEMIA

Recurrent antecedent hypoglycemia induces impaired sympathoadrenal responses and hypoglycemia unawareness. Fortunately, avoidance of hypoglycemia can completely restore hypoglycemia awareness, and partially restore the adrenomedullary response to hypoglycemia.[104–106] Studies showed an improved awareness after 3 days, and normalized hypoglycemia awareness with improved evidence of counterregulation after as little as 3 weeks of hypoglycemia avoidance. Thus, the adaptations that occur in response to recurrent hypoglycemia are reversible. As hypoglycemia begets hypoglycemia, so does hypoglycemia avoidance avoid hypoglycemia.

PATIENT EDUCATION

There are 2 types of patient-education strategies that aim to decrease the incidence of hypoglycemia. Psychological-based instructional programs aim to improve the patients' accuracy in detecting hypoglycemia.[107,108] Other educational programs advocate hypoglycemia avoidance strategies, dietary education, and flexible insulin-dosing strategies to account for varied diet and activity levels.[109,110] Efficacy of these educational programs is noteworthy. In the setting of intensified control of blood glucose (reducing HbA1c from 8.1% to 7.3%), when rates of hypoglycemia would be expected to increase, educational programs markedly reduced the incidence of severe hypoglycemia from 0.37 to 0.14 events per patient per year.[110] Thus, patient education seems to break the bond that hitherto invariably linked intensive glycemic control to increased incidence of hypoglycemia.

CHOICE OF INSULIN ANALOGUE THERAPY

Multiple clinical trials demonstrate that the newer insulin analogues reduce the incidence of hypoglycemia. With a shorter duration of action compared with regular insulin, rapid-acting insulin analogues decrease the incidence of postprandial hypoglycemia.[111,112] By not rising in the middle of the night, the flatter pharmacokinetics of long-acting insulin glargine help to decrease the incidence of nocturnal hypoglycemia in comparison with NPH insulin.[113] The newer ultra–long-acting basal insulin degludec appears to be particularly effective in lowering the risk of nocturnal hypoglycemia.[114]

CHOICE OF INSULIN DELIVERY: USE OF CONTINUOUS SUBCUTANEOUS INSULIN INFUSION PUMPS

If an HbA1c of less than 8.5% is not obtainable via multiple doses of injectable insulin, a clinical decision to initiate a trial of a continuous subcutaneous insulin infusion (CSII) pump is reasonable. A review analysis of 26 observational studies noted that most CSII studies demonstrated significantly decreased rates of severe hypoglycemia.[115] A recent prospective study specifically recruiting patients with hypoglycemia unawareness showed that transitioning patients from multiple daily injections to CSII halved the hypoglycemic events rate and, remarkably, virtually eliminated the rate of severe hypoglycemia, from 1.25 to 0.05 events per year.[116] Thus, the use of CSII may reduce the amount of human error that occurs with multiple daily insulin injections and thereby reduce episodes of hypoglycemia.

SELF-MONITORING OF BLOOD GLUCOSE: CONTINUOUS GLUCOSE MONITORS

A meta-analysis of 19 trials indicated that continuous glucose monitors (CGM) improve glycemic control in adults with diabetes but, despite hypoglycemia alarms, the effect on reducing the incidence of hypoglycemia is marginal.[117] A more positive interpretation would be that the use of CGM improves HbA1c without increasing the incidence of hypoglycemia,[118] results very much unlike the Diabetes Control and Complications Trial.[3] Therefore, CGM technology may help dissociate intensive glycemic control from increased hypoglycemia.

Establishing closed-loop communication between CGM and insulin pumps may offer new technology-based opportunities to decrease the burden of hypoglycemia. For example, programming of insulin pumps to automatically suspend basal insulin infusion for 2 hours after a low blood-sugar level detected by CGM significantly decreases the duration of hypoglycemia.[119] In addition to suspending insulin delivery, perhaps technology in the near future will allow dual-chamber pumps to automatically infuse glucagon in response to a low or falling blood-glucose level to limit the incidence, duration, or severity of hypoglycemia.[120]

WHOLE PANCREAS AND ISLET CELL TRANSPLANTATION

Continuous glucose monitoring systems have confirmed that transplant recipients either have significantly decreased (in insulin-requiring subjects) or completely eradicated (in insulin-independent subjects) the amount of time spent in the hypoglycemic range (<60 mg/dL).[121] The mechanisms for this striking reduction in the incidence of hypoglycemia include (1) the elimination (or marked reduction) in exogenous insulin administration, which reduces the risk of iatrogenic hypoglycemia; (2) the provision of a regulatory decrement in endogenous insulin secretion; (3) the partial restoration of the glucagon CRR; and (4) the recovery of sympathoadrenal response and hypoglycemia awareness owing to the avoidance of iatrogenic hypoglycemia.[122,123] For patients with intractable, recurrent, severe hypoglycemia, transplantation of whole pancreas or islet cells should be considered as a viable therapeutic option.

RELAXED HBA1C GOALS

Although the American Diabetes Association and the American Association of Clinical Endocrinologists differ with regard to HbA1c goals (<7.0% or ≤6.5%, respectively), both societies acknowledge that these goals should only be attempted if they can be achieved safely "without significant/substantial hypoglycemia." Given that significant/substantial, temporarily disabling, severe hypoglycemia occurs so frequently in people with both type 1 and type 2 diabetes,[8] it could be argued that these idyllic HbA1c goals

---

Box 1
Clinical indications for less strict HbA1c goals (ie, goal HbA1c in 7%–8% range)

Advanced age

Pediatric patients

Hypoglycemia unawareness

Frequent severe hypoglycemia

Life expectancy less than 5 years

Advanced macrovascular complications

Renal failure

Extensive comorbidities

Table 1
Recommended review of hypoglycemia at clinic visits

Monitoring	Recent history of symptomatic or severe hypoglycemia
	Recent history of hypoglycemia unawareness
	Recommend frequent blood-glucose measurements
	Monitor carbohydrate intake and insulin dosage, special events/considerations
	Review data: assess for patterns of hypoglycemia (time of day, association with types of meals/activities/exercise, weekdays vs weekends, postmenstrual)
	Recommend checking blood sugar before meals, at bedtime, and before driving
	Consider referral for diabetes education
	If nocturnal hypoglycemia is suspected, wake patient at 3 AM for a few nights to check blood glucose
	Consideration of a continuous glucose-monitoring system with hypoglycemia alarms
Meals	Adjust insulin-to-carbohydrate ratio to avoid postmeal hypoglycemia
	Proper assessment of portion size and carbohydrate content
	Ideal insulin-to-carbohydrate ratio should reach target blood sugar 3 to 4 h after meals
	Premeal glycemia may influence the timing delay between premeal insulin dosage and initiating of meal
	If premeal glucose is below target, reduce premeal insulin dose appropriately
	Alcohol has glucose-lowering effects and can mask symptoms of hypoglycemia; consider reducing basal insulin doses when consuming alcohol
Insulin	Insulin basal long-acting + rapid-acting premeal insulin combinations less likely to cause hypoglycemia than intermediate-acting + regular insulin preparations
	Consider less aggressive correction insulin doses. Use the 1800 Rule rather than the 1500 Rule (ie, estimated mg/dL drop in glycemia per unit of insulin = 1800/total daily dose)
	Avoid repetitive, or stacking of, correction doses
Exercise	Consider type of exercise (timing, duration, and intensity)
	Check blood sugars before and during prolonged exercise; snack if necessary
	Consider reducing basal insulin dosage before anticipated period of prolonged exercise
	Make adjustments for increased insulin sensitivity for 24 h after exercise
Treatment	Readily available emergency supplies including sugar tablets, candy, sugar-paste in tube
	Prescription glucagon kits (nonexpired) readily available
	People who have regular contact with patient (family members, colleagues, teachers, etc) need to know signs of hypoglycemia and how to treat it
	Notification of emergency medical services (ie, 911)
Prevention	Discussion between patient and physician regarding a period of less intensive glycemic management goals (ie, relaxed/higher glycated hemoglobin goal, higher blood-glucose targets pre/post meals, when calculating correction factor, etc)
	Review comorbidities that cause hypoglycemia including malabsorption (celiac or pancreatic insufficiency), renal failure, liver disease, adrenal insufficiency, hypothyroidism
	Scrupulous avoidance of hypoglycemia to restore hypoglycemia awareness
	Medical identification bracelet or necklace indicating that patient has diabetes and takes insulin

Table 2
Investigational and advanced therapies for hypoglycemia prevention

Interventions	Rational	Reference

Bedtime Snacks
  Carbohydrate/protein
  Carbohydrate/protein + acarbose
  Uncooked cornstarch bars
	Prevention of early nocturnal hypoglycemia	125,126

Insulin pump and continuous glucose monitors
  Automatic basal insulin suspension
  Dual-chamber insulin and glucagon pumps
	Prevention of iatrogenic insulin–induced hypoglycemia	120,127

Alert dogs	Dogs trained to recognize hypoglycemia and alert owners	128
Islet cell or whole pancreas transplantation	Restoration of the counterregulatory response	122,123

Medications
  Theophylline
  Caffeine
  Terbutaline
  Fluoxetine
	Increase hypoglycemic counterregulatory response and patient perception of hypoglycemia	125,129,130

are not appropriate for a relatively large percentage of people with diabetes. To decrease the incidence of hypoglycemia, both societies advocate less stringent HbA1c goals (such as 8%) as being appropriate for patients with a history of severe hypoglycemia. Also, for young children who are often unable to recognize the symptoms of hypoglycemia, relaxed glycemic control guidelines are recommended (**Box 1**).[124] In addition, relaxed HbA1c goals may be appropriate for patients in whom one severe hypoglycemic reaction might be particularly catastrophic (ie, frail elderly people with diabetes, patients with extensive comorbid conditions or advanced macrovascular complications). Finally, less strict HbA1c goals may be appropriate for individuals in whom the benefits of intensive glycemic control may not be realized (ie, patients with advanced microvascular complications or limited life expectancy). Therefore, ideal HbA1c target goals should not be generalized for all individuals with diabetes; rather, health care practitioners should individualize realistic HbA1c goals on a case-by-case basis to minimize the potential morbidity and mortality of hypoglycemia.

SUMMARY

Until a cure for diabetes is found, hypoglycemia will continue to be a major barrier for the achievement of long-term glucose control and will cause recurrent morbidity in individuals with diabetes (**Tables 1** and **2**). Numerous sedulous research studies have begun to uncover the mechanisms by which the CNS responds and adapts to hypoglycemia. Understanding these mechanisms will undoubtedly lead to better management and therapies that reduce the risk for hypoglycemia, while still allowing patients to achieve the benefits associated with tight glycemic control. Given this pervasive barrier of hypoglycemia for the treatment of diabetes, physicians should discuss hypoglycemia prevention strategies with their patients, so that they can have a better chance of achieving their glucose controls goals while avoiding the morbidity and mortality associated with hypoglycemia.

REFERENCES

1. Duckworth W, Abraira C, Moritz T, et al. Glucose control and vascular complications in veterans with type 2 diabetes. N Engl J Med 2009;360:129–39.
2. Terry T, Raravikar K, Chokrungvaranon N, et al. Does aggressive glycemic control benefit macrovascular and microvascular disease in type 2 diabetes? Insights from ACCORD, ADVANCE, and VADT. Curr Cardiol Rep 2012;14:79–88.
3. The Diabetes Control and Complications Trial Research Group. The effect of intensive treatment of diabetes on the development and progression of long-term complications in insulin-dependent diabetes mellitus. N Engl J Med 1993;329:977–96.
4. Turner RC, Holman RR, Stratton IM, et al. Effect of intensive blood-glucose control with metformin on complications in overweight patients with type 2 diabetes (UKPDS 34). Lancet 1998;352:854–65.
5. The ADVANCE collaborative group. Intensive blood glucose control and vascular outcomes in patients with type 2 diabetes. N Engl J Med 2008;358:2560–72.
6. Kubiak T, Hermanns N, Schreckling HJ, et al. Assessment of hypoglycaemia awareness using continuous glucose monitoring. Diabet Med 2004;21:487–90.
7. Cryer PE. Hypoglycemia-associated autonomic failure in diabetes. Am J Physiol Endocrinol Metab 2001;281:E1115–21.
8. Heller SR, Choudhary P, Davies C, et al. Risk of hypoglycaemia in types 1 and 2 diabetes: effects of treatment modalities and their duration. Diabetologia 2007; 50:1140–7.
9. Perantie DC, Wu J, Koller JM, et al. Regional brain volume differences associated with hyperglycemia and severe hypoglycemia in youth with type 1 diabetes. Diabetes Care 2007;30:2331–7.
10. Suh SW, Hamby AM, Swanson RA. Hypoglycemia, brain energetics, and hypoglycemic neuronal death. Glia 2007;55:1280–6.
11. Puente EC, Silverstein J, Bree AJ, et al. Recurrent moderate hypoglycemia ameliorates brain damage and cognitive dysfunction induced by severe hypoglycemia. Diabetes 2010;59:1055–62.
12. Northam EA, Rankins D, Lin A, et al. Central nervous system function in youth with type 1 diabetes 12 years after disease onset. Diabetes Care 2009;32:445–50.
13. Asvold BO, Sand T, Hestad K, et al. Cognitive function in type 1 diabetic adults with early exposure to severe hypoglycemia: a 16-year follow-up study. Diabetes Care 2010;33:1945–7.
14. Tanenberg RJ, Newton CA, Drake AJ. Confirmation of hypoglycemia in the "dead-in-bed" syndrome, as captured by a retrospective continuous glucose monitoring system. Endocr Pathol 2010;16:244–8.
15. Feltbower RG, Bodansky HJ, Patterson CC, et al. Acute complications and drug misuse are important causes of death for children and young adults with type 1 diabetes - Results from the Yorkshire Register of Diabetes in Children and Young Adults. Diabetes Care 2008;31:922–6.
16. Jacobson AM, Musen G, Ryan CM, et al. Long-term effect of diabetes and its treatment on cognitive function. N Engl J Med 2007;356:1842–52.
17. Skrivarhaug T, Bangstad HJ, Stene LC, et al. Long-term mortality in a nationwide cohort of childhood-onset type 1 diabetic patients in Norway. Diabetologia 2006; 49:298–305.
18. Reno CM, Daphna-Iken D, Fisher SJ. Adrenergic blockade prevents life threatening cardiac arrhythmias and sudden death due to severe hypoglycemia. Diabetes 2012;61:A46.

19. Frier BM, Schernthaner G, Heller SR. Hypoglycemia and cardiovascular risks. Diabetes Care 2011;34:S132–7.
20. Segel SA, Paramore DS, Cryer PE. Hypoglycemia-associated autonomic failure in advanced type 2 diabetes. Diabetes 2002;51:724–33.
21. Cryer PE. Minireview: glucagon in the pathogenesis of hypoglycemia and hyperglycemia in diabetes. Endocrinology 2012;153:1039–48.
22. Taborsky GJ, Mundinger TO. Minireview: the role of the autonomic nervous system in mediating the glucagon response to hypoglycemia. Endocrinology 2012;153:1055–62.
23. Yue JT, Burdett E, Coy DH, et al. Somatostatin receptor type 2 antagonism improves glucagon and corticosterone counterregulatory responses to hypoglycemia in streptozotocin-induced diabetic rats. Diabetes 2012;61:197–207.
24. DeRosa MA, Cryer PE. Hypoglycemia and the sympathoadrenal system: neurogenic symptoms are largely the result of sympathetic neural, rather than adrenomedullary, activation. Am J Physiol Endocrinol Metab 2004;287:E32–41.
25. Zammitt NN, Streftaris G, Gibson GJ, et al. Modeling the consistency of hypoglycemic symptoms: high variability in diabetes. Diabetes Technol Ther 2011;13:571–8.
26. Mitrakou A, Ryan C, Veneman T, et al. Hierarchy of glycemic thresholds for counterregulatory hormone-secretion, symptoms, and cerebral-dysfunction. Am J Physiol 1991;260:E67–74.
27. Borg MA, Borg WP, Tamborlane WV, et al. Chronic hypoglycemia and diabetes impair counterregulation induced by localized 2-deoxy-glucose perfusion of the ventromedial hypothalamus in rats. Diabetes 1999;48:584–7.
28. Tong QC, Ye CP, McCrimmon RJ, et al. Synaptic glutamate release by ventromedial hypothalamic neurons is part of the neurocircuitry that prevents hypoglycemia. Cell Metab 2007;5:383–93.
29. Page KA, Arora J, Qiu M, et al. Small decrements in systemic glucose provoke increases in hypothalamic blood flow prior to the release of counterregulatory hormones. Diabetes 2009;58:448–52.
30. Watts AG, Donovan CM. Sweet talk in the brain: glucosensing, neural networks, and hypoglycemic counterregulation. Front Neuroendocrinol 2010;31:32–43.
31. Borg MA, Sherwin RS, Borg WP, et al. Local ventromedial hypothalamus glucose perfusion blocks counterregulation during systemic hypoglycemia in awake rats. J Clin Invest 1997;99:361–5.
32. de Vries MG, Lawson MA, Beverly JL. Hypoglycemia-induced noradrenergic activation in the VMH is a result of decreased ambient glucose. Am J Physiol Regul Integr Comp Physiol 2005;289:R977–81.
33. Kang L, Routh VH, Kuzhikandathil EV, et al. Physiological and molecular characteristics of rat hypothalamic ventromedial nucleus glucosensing neurons. Diabetes 2004;53:549–59.
34. Routh VH. Glucose sensing neurons in the ventromedial hypothalamus. Sensors (Basel) 2010;10:9002–25.
35. Medeiros N, Dai L, Ferguson AV. Glucose-responsive neurons in the subfornical organ of the rat–a novel site for direct CNS monitoring of circulating glucose. Neuroscience 2012;201:157–65.
36. Dallaporta M, Himmi T, Perrin J, et al. Solitary tract nucleus sensitivity to moderate changes in glucose level. Neuroreport 1999;10:2657–60.

37. Shapiro RE, Miselis RR. The central neural connections of the area postrema of the rat. J Comp Neurol 1985;234:344–64.
38. Paranjape SA, Briski KP. Recurrent insulin-induced hypoglycemia causes site-specific patterns of habituation or amplification of CNS neuronal genomic activation. Neuroscience 2005;130:957–70.
39. Diggs-Andrews KA, Zhang X, Song Z, et al. Brain insulin action regulates hypothalamic glucose sensing and the counterregulatory response to hypoglycemia. Diabetes 2010;59:2271–80.
40. Marty N, Dallaporta M, Foretz M, et al. Regulation of glucagon secretion by glucose transporter type 2 (glut2) and astrocyte-dependent glucose sensors. J Clin Invest 2005;115:3545–53.
41. Puente E, Daphna-Iken D, Bree AJ, et al. Impaired counterregulatory response to hypoglycemia and impaired glucose tolerance in brain glucose transporter 4 (GLUT4) knockout mice [abstract]. Diabetes 2009;58(Suppl):A13.
42. Dunn-Meynell AA, Routh VH, Kang L, et al. Glucokinase is the likely mediator of glucosensing in both glucose-excited and glucose-inhibited central neurons. Diabetes 2002;51:2056–65.
43. Levin BE, Becker TC, Eiki J, et al. Ventromedial hypothalamic glucokinase is an important mediator of the counterregulatory response to insulin-induced hypoglycemia. Diabetes 2008;57:1371–9.
44. McCrimmon RJ, Shaw M, Fan XN, et al. Key role for AMP-activated protein kinase in the ventromedial hypothalamus in regulating counterregulatory hormone responses to acute hypoglycemia. Diabetes 2008;57:444–50.
45. Fioramonti X, Marsollier N, Song ZT, et al. Ventromedial hypothalamic nitric oxide production is necessary for hypoglycemia detection and counterregulation. Diabetes 2010;59:519–28.
46. McCrimmon RJ, Evans ML, Fan XN, et al. Activation of ATP-sensitive K^+ channels in the ventromedial hypothalamus amplifies counterregulatory hormone responses to hypoglycemia in normal and recurrently hypoglycemic rats. Diabetes 2005;54:3169–74.
47. Spanswick D, Smith MA, Mirshamsi S, et al. Insulin activates ATP-sensitive K^+ channels in hypothalamic neurons of lean, but not obese rats. Nat Neurosci 2000;3:757–8.
48. Davis SN, Colburn C, Dobbins R, et al. Evidence that the brain of the conscious dog is insulin-sensitive. J Clin Invest 1995;95:593–602.
49. Beverly JL, De Vries MG, Bouman SD, et al. Noradrenergic and GABAergic systems in the medial hypothalamus are activated during hypoglycemia. Am J Physiol Regul Integr Comp Physiol 2001;280:R563–9.
50. Barnes MB, Lawson MA, Beverly JL. Rate of fall in blood glucose and recurrent hypoglycemia affect glucose dynamics and noradrenergic activation in the ventromedial hypothalamus. Am J Physiol Regul Integr Comp Physiol 2011;301:R1815–20.
51. Szepietowska B, Zhu WL, Chan OW, et al. Modulation of beta-adrenergic receptors in the ventromedial hypothalamus influences counterregulatory responses to hypoglycemia. Diabetes 2011;60:3154–8.
52. Saberi M, Bohland M, Donovan CM. The locus for hypoglycemic rate of fall in glycemia—the role of portal-superior mesenteric vein glucose sensing. Diabetes 2008;57:1380–6.
53. Cryer PE. Elimination of hypoglycemia from the lives of people affected by diabetes. Diabetes 2011;60:24–7.

54. Cryer PE. Hypoglycaemia: the limiting factor in the glycaemic management of type I and type II diabetes. Diabetologia 2002;45:937–48.

55. Song ZT, Routh VH. Recurrent hypoglycemia reduces the glucose sensitivity of glucose-inhibited neurons in the ventromedial hypothalamus nucleus. Am J Physiol Regul Integr Comp Physiol 2006;291:R1283–7.

56. Geddes J, Schopman JE, Zammitt NN, et al. Prevalence of impaired awareness of hypoglycaemia in adults with type 1 diabetes. Diabet Med 2008;25:501–4.

57. Schopman JE, Geddes J, Frier BM. Prevalence of impaired awareness of hypoglycaemia and frequency of hypoglycaemia in insulin-treated type 2 diabetes. Diabetes Res Clin Pract 2010;87:64–8.

58. McCrimmon RJ, Sherwin RS. Hypoglycemia in type 1 diabetes. Diabetes 2010;59:2333–9.

59. McCrimmon RJ, Song ZT, Cheng HY, et al. Corticotrophin-releasing factor receptors within the ventromedial hypothalamus regulate hypoglycemia-induced hormonal counterregulation. J Clin Invest 2006;116:1723–30.

60. McGregor VP, Banarer S, Cryer PE. Elevated endogenous cortisol reduces autonomic neuroendocrine and symptom responses to subsequent hypoglycemia. Am J Physiol Endocrinol Metab 2002;282:E770–7.

61. Davis SN, Shavers C, Davis B, et al. Prevention of an increase in plasma cortisol during hypoglycemia preserves subsequent counterregulatory responses. J Clin Invest 1997;100:429–38.

62. Davis SN, Shavers C, Costa F, et al. Role of cortisol in the pathogenesis of deficient counterregulation after antecedent hypoglycemia in normal humans. J Clin Invest 1996;98:680–91.

63. Raju B, McGregor VP, Cryer PE. Cortisol elevations comparable to those that occur during hypoglycemia do not cause hypoglycemia-associated autonomic failure. Diabetes 2003;52:2083–9.

64. Goldberg PA, Weiss R, McCrimmon RJ, et al. Antecedent hypercortisolemia is not primarily responsible for generating hypoglycemia-associated autonomic failure. Diabetes 2006;55:1121–6.

65. Ramanathan R, Cryer PE. Adrenergic mediation of hypoglycemia-associated autonomic failure. Diabetes 2011;60:602–6.

66. Caprio S, Gerety G, Tamborlane WV, et al. Opiate blockade enhances hypoglycemic counterregulation in normal and insulin-dependent diabetic subjects. Am J Physiol 1991;260:E852–8.

67. Vele S, Milman S, Shamoon H, et al. Opioid receptor blockade improves hypoglycemia-associated autonomic failure in type 1 diabetes mellitus. J Clin Endocrinol Metab 2011;96:3424–31.

68. Poplawski MM, Mastaitis JW, Mobbs CV. Naloxone, but not Valsartan, preserves responses to hypoglycemia after antecedent hypoglycemia role of metabolic reprogramming in counterregulatory failure. Diabetes 2011;60:39–46.

69. Galassetti P, Mann S, Tate D, et al. Effects of antecedent prolonged exercise on subsequent counterregulatory responses to hypoglycemia. Am J Physiol Endocrinol Metab 2001;280:E908–17.

70. Milman S, Leu J, Shamoon H, et al. Magnitude of exercise-induced beta-endorphin response is associated with subsequent development of altered hypoglycemia counterregulation. J Clin Endocrinol Metab 2012;97:623–31.

71. Ahmet A, Dagenais S, Barrowman NJ, et al. Prevalence of nocturnal hypoglycemia in pediatric type 1 diabetes: a pilot study using continuous glucose monitoring. J Pediatr 2011;159:297–U385.

72. Wiltshire EJ, Newton K, McTavish L. Unrecognised hypoglycaemia in children and adolescents with type 1 diabetes using the continuous glucose monitoring system: prevalence and contributors. J Paediatr Child Health 2006;42:758–63.

73. Jones TW, Porter P, Sherwin RS, et al. Decreased epinephrine responses to hypoglycemia during sleep. N Engl J Med 1998;338:1657–62.

74. Banarer S, Cryer PE. Sleep-related hypoglycemia-associated autonomic failure in type 1 diabetes—reduced awakening from sleep during hypoglycemia. Diabetes 2003;52:1195–203.

75. Tattersall RB, Gill GV. Unexplained deaths of type 1 diabetic patients. Diabet Med 1991;8:49–58.

76. Oz G, Kumar A, Rao JP, et al. Human brain glycogen metabolism during and after hypoglycemia. Diabetes 2009;58:1978–85.

77. Canada SE, Weaver SA, Sharpe SN, et al. Brain glycogen supercompensation in the mouse after recovery from insulin-induced hypoglycemia. J Neurosci Res 2011;89:585–91.

78. Alquier T, Kawashima J, Tsuji Y, et al. Role of hypothalamic adenosine 5'-monophosphate activated protein kinase in the impaired counterregulatory response induced by repetitive neuroglucopenia. Endocrinology 2007;148:1367–75.

79. Herzog RI, Chan O, Yu S, et al. Effect of acute and recurrent hypoglycemia on changes in brain glycogen concentration. Endocrinology 2008;149:1499–504.

80. Oz G, Tesfaye N, Kumar A, et al. Brain glycogen content and metabolism in subjects with type 1 diabetes and hypoglycemia unawareness. J Cereb Blood Flow Metab 2012;32:256–63.

81. Mastaitis JW, Wurmbach E, Cheng H, et al. Acute induction of gene expression in brain and liver by insulin-induced hypoglycemia. Diabetes 2005;54: 952–8.

82. Koranyi L, Bourey RE, James D, et al. Glucose transporter gene expression in rat brain: pretranslational changes associated with chronic insulin-induced hypoglycemia, fasting, and diabetes. Mol Cell Neurosci 1991;2:244–52.

83. Osundiji MA, Hurst P, Moore SP, et al. Recurrent hypoglycemia increases hypothalamic glucose phosphorylation activity in rats. Metabolism 2011;60:550–6.

84. Jiang LH, Herzog RI, Mason GF, et al. Recurrent antecedent hypoglycemia alters neuronal oxidative metabolism in vivo. Diabetes 2009;58:1266–74.

85. van de Ven KC, van der Graaf M, Tack CJ, et al. Steady-state brain glucose concentrations during hypoglycemia in healthy humans and patients with type 1 diabetes mellitus. Diabetes 2012;61(8):1974–7.

86. Cranston I, Reed LJ, Marsden PK, et al. Changes in regional brain (18)F-fluorodeoxyglucose uptake at hypoglycemia in type 1 diabetic men associated with hypoglycemia unawareness and counter-regulatory failure. Diabetes 2001;50: 2329–36.

87. Bingham EM, Dunn JT, Smith D, et al. Differential changes in brain glucose metabolism during hypoglycaemia accompany loss of hypoglycaemia awareness in men with type 1 diabetes mellitus. An [C-11]-3-O-methyl-D-glucose PET study. Diabetologia 2005;48:2080–9.

88. Dunn JT, Cranston I, Marsden PK, et al. Attenuation of amygdala and frontal cortical responses to low blood glucose concentration in asymptomatic hypoglycemia in type 1 diabetes—a new player in hypoglycemia unawareness? Diabetes 2007;56:2766–73.

89. Segel SA, Fanelli CG, Dence CS, et al. Blood-to-brain glucose transport, cerebral glucose metabolism, and cerebral blood flow are not increased after hypoglycemia. Diabetes 2001;50:1911–7.

90. Arbelaez AM, Powers WJ, Videen TO, et al. Attenuation of counterregulatory responses to recurrent hypoglycemia by active thalamic inhibition—a mechanism for hypoglycemia-associated autonomic failure. Diabetes 2008;57:470–5.

91. Herzog RI, Jiang L, Mason G, et al. Increased brain lactate utilization following exposure to recurrent hypoglycemia. Diabetes 2009;58:A14.

92. Mason GF, Petersen KF, Lebon V, et al. Increased brain monocarboxylic acid transport and utilization in type 1 diabetes. Diabetes 2006;55:929–34.

93. Feyter HD, Shulman G, Rothman D, et al. Increased brain uptake of lactate in type I diabetic patients with hypoglycemia unawareness. Diabetes 2012;61:A33.

94. Oz G, Moheet A, Emir U, et al. Hypothalamic GABA drops in response to acute hypoglycemia in healthy humans. Diabetes 2012;61:A32.

95. Chan O, Paranjape S, Czyzyk D, et al. Increased GABAergic output in the ventromedial hypothalamus contributes to impaired hypoglycemic counterregulation in diabetic rats. Diabetes 2011;60:1582–9.

96. Chan O, Cheng HY, Herzog R, et al. Increased GABAergic tone in the ventromedial hypothalamus contributes to suppression of counterregulatory responses after antecedent hypoglycemia. Diabetes 2008;57:1363–70.

97. Boyle PJ, Nagy RJ, O'Connor AM, et al. Adaptation in brain glucose uptake following recurrent hypoglycemia. Proc Natl Acad Sci U S A 1994;91:9352–6.

98. Reno CM, Tanoli T, Puente EC, et al. Deaths due to severe hypoglycemia are exacerbated by diabetes and ameliorated by hypoglycemic preconditioning. Diabetes 2011;60:A81.

99. Smith CB, Choudhary P, Pernet A, et al. Hypoglycemia unawareness is associated with reduced adherence to therapeutic decisions in patients with type 1 diabetes evidence from a clinical audit. Diabetes Care 2009;32:1196–8.

100. Matyka K, Evans M, Lomas J, et al. Altered hierarchy of protective responses against severe hypoglycemia in normal aging in healthy men. Diabetes Care 1997;20:135–41.

101. Davis SN, Shavers C, Costa F. Gender-related differences in counterregulatory responses to antecedent hypoglycemia in normal humans. J Clin Endocrinol Metab 2000;85:2148–57.

102. Sandoval DA, Ertl AC, Richardson MA, et al. Estrogen blunts neuroendocrine and metabolic responses to hypoglycemia. Diabetes 2003;52:1749–55.

103. McGill JB, Vlajnic A, Knutsen PG, et al. Effect of gender on outcomes in patients with T2DM treated with insulin glargine vs comparators. Diabetes 2011;60:A602.

104. Dagogo-Jack S, Rattarasarn C, Cryer PE. Reversal of hypoglycemia unawareness, but not defective glucose counterregulation, in IDDM. Diabetes 1994;43:1426–34.

105. Cranston I, Lomas J, Maran A, et al. Restoration of hypoglycemia awareness in patients with long-duration insulin-dependent diabetes. Lancet 1994;344:283–7.

106. Fanelli CG, Epifano L, Rambotti AM, et al. Meticulous prevention of hypoglycemia normalizes the glycemic thresholds and magnitude of most of neuroendocrine responses to, symptoms of, and cognitive function during hypoglycemia in intensively treated patients with short-term IDDM. Diabetes 1993;42:1683–9.

107. Cox DJ, Gonder-Frederick L, Polonsky W, et al. Blood glucose awareness training (BGAT-2)—long-term benefits. Diabetes Care 2001;24:637–42.

108. Cox DJ, Kovatchev B, Koev D, et al. Hypoglycemia anticipation, awareness and treatment training (HAATT) reduces occurrence of severe hypoglycemia among adults with type 1 diabetes mellitus. Int J Behav Med 2004;11:212–8.

109. Hopkins D, Lawrence I, Mansell P, et al. Improved biomedical and psychological outcomes 1 year after structured education in flexible insulin therapy for people with type 1 diabetes the U.K. DAFNE experience. Diabetes Care 2012;35: 1638–42.
110. Samann A, Muhlhauser I, Bender R, et al. Glycaemic control and severe hypo-glycaemia following training in flexible, intensive insulin therapy to enable die-tary freedom in people with type 1 diabetes: a prospective implementation study. Diabetologia 2005;48:1965–70.
111. Heller SR, Colagiuri S, Vaaler S, et al. Hypoglycaemia with insulin aspart: a double-blind, randomised, crossover trial in subjects with type 1 diabetes. Diabet Med 2004;21:769–75.
112. Brunelle RL, Llewelyn J, Anderson JH, et al. Meta-analysis of the effect of insulin lispro on severe hypoglycemia in patients with type 1 diabetes. Diabetes Care 1998;21:1726–31.
113. Home PD, Fritsche A, Schinzel S, et al. Meta-analysis of individual patient data to assess the risk of hypoglycaemia in people with type 2 diabetes using NPH insulin or insulin glargine. Diabetes Obes Metab 2010;12:772–9.
114. Heller S, Buse J, Fisher M, et al. Insulin degludec, an ultra-long-acting basal insulin, versus insulin glargine in basal-bolus treatment with mealtime insulin as-part in type 1 diabetes (BEGIN Basal-Bolus Type 1): a phase 3, randomised, open-label, treat-to-target non-inferiority trial. Lancet 2012;379:1489–97.
115. Cummins E, Royle P, Snaith A, et al. Clinical effectiveness and cost-effectiveness of continuous subcutaneous insulin infusion for diabetes: system-atic review and economic evaluation. Health Technol Assess 2010;14(11):iii–iiv.
116. Gimenez M, Lara M, Conget I. Sustained efficacy of continuous subcutaneous insulin infusion in type 1 diabetes subjects with recurrent non-severe and severe hypoglycemia and hypoglycemia unawareness: a pilot study. Diabetes Technol Ther 2010;12:517–21.
117. Gandhi GY, Kovalaske M, Kudva Y, et al. Efficacy of continuous glucose moni-toring in improving glycemic control and reducing hypoglycemia: a systematic review and meta-analysis of randomized trials. J Diabetes Sci Technol 2011;5: 952–65.
118. Juvenile Diabetes Research Foundation Continuous Glucose Monitoring Study Group, Beck RW, Hirsch IB, et al. The effect of continuous glucose monitoring in well-controlled type 1 diabetes. Diabetes Care 2009;32:1378–83.
119. Garg S, Brazg RL, Bailey TS, et al. Reduction in duration of hypoglycemia by automatic suspension of insulin delivery: the in-clinic ASPIRE study. Diabetes Technol Ther 2012;14:205–9.
120. El-Khatib FH, Russell SJ, Nathan DM, et al. A bihormonal closed-loop artificial pancreas for type 1 diabetes. Sci Transl Med 2010;2:27ra27.
121. Paty BW, Senior PA, Lakey JRT, et al. Assessment of glycemic control after islet transplantation using the continuous glucose monitor in insulin-independent versus insulin-requiring type 1 diabetes subjects. Diabetes Technol Ther 2006;8:165–73.
122. Leitao CB, Tharavanij T, Cure P, et al. Restoration of hypoglycemia awareness after islet transplantation. Diabetes Care 2008;31:2113–5.
123. Rickels MR. Recovery of endocrine function after islet and pancreas transplan-tation. Curr Diab Rep 2012;12(5):587–96.
124. Silverstein J, Klingensmith G, Copeland K, et al. Care of children and adoles-cents with type 1 diabetes: a statement of the American Diabetes Association. Diabetes Care 2005;28:186–212.

125. Raju B, Arbelaez AM, Breckenridge SM, et al. Nocturnal hypoglycemia in type 1 diabetes: an assessment of preventive bedtime treatments. J Clin Endocrinol Metab 2006;91:2087–92.

126. Axelsen M, Wesslau C, Lonnroth P, et al. Bedtime uncooked cornstarch supplement prevents nocturnal hypoglycaemia in intensively treated type 1 diabetes subjects. J Intern Med 1999;245:229–36.

127. Weinzimer SA. Closed-loop artificial pancreas: current studies and promise for the future. Curr Opin Endocrinol Diabetes Obes 2012;19:88–92.

128. Hardin D, Hillman D, Cattet J. Hypoglycemia alert dogs—innovative assistance for people with type I diabetes. Diabetes 2012;61:A99.

129. Watson JM, Jenkins EE, Hamilton P, et al. Influence of caffeine on the frequency and perception at hypoglycemia in free-living patients with type 1 diabetes. Diabetes Care 2000;23:455–9.

130. de Galan BE, Tack CJ, Lenders JW, et al. Effect of 2 weeks of theophylline on glucose counterregulation in patients with type 1 diabetes and unawareness of hypoglycemia. Clin Pharmacol Ther 2003;74:77–84.

Novel Approaches to Studying the Role of Innervation in the Biology of Pancreatic Islets

Rayner Rodriguez-Diaz, PhD[a],*, Alejandro Caicedo, PhD[a,b,c,d],*

KEYWORDS

- Innervation • Pancreas • Islet cells • Islets of Langerhans

KEY POINTS

- Studying the functional role of autonomic innervation in pancreatic islet function is difficult.
- Recent advances in microscopy and novel approaches to studying the effects of nervous input may help clarify how autonomic axons regulate islet biology.

INTRODUCTION

A well-functioning endocrine pancreas, the islets of Langerhans, is crucial for survival. The islets of Langerhans secrete hormones that maintain constant levels of plasma glucose. Dysfunction or death of the insulin-secreting β cells leads to potentially life-threatening fluctuations in plasma glucose levels and is a major cause of diabetes mellitus, a devastating disease affecting millions worldwide. In the nineteenth century, Claude Bernard[1] proposed that the nervous system is implicated in the regulation of plasma glucose and since their discovery Langerhans[2] recognized a rich innervation of the islets. Many studies have linked the autonomic nervous system to metabolic control and islet function.[3–8] However, the importance of the autonomic innervation of the islets in the maintenance of glucose homeostasis has remained controversial for 2 main reasons: (1) there is a lack of detailed anatomic studies of islet innervation,

Funding sources: Diabetes Research Institute Foundation, NIH grants R56DK084321 and R01DK084321.
Conflict of interest: A.C. holds a patent on the use of the anterior chamber of the eye as a commercial servicing platform.
[a] Diabetes Research Institute, Miller School of Medicine, University of Miami, Miami, FL 33136, USA; [b] Department of Medicine, Miller School of Medicine, University of Miami, 1580 Northwest 10th Avenue, Miami, FL 33136, USA; [c] Department of Physiology and Biophysics, Miller School of Medicine, University of Miami, Miami, FL 33136, USA; [d] Program in Neuroscience, Miller School of Medicine, University of Miami, Miami, FL 33136, USA
* Corresponding authors. Department of Medicine, Miller School of Medicine, University of Miami, 1580 Northwest 10th Avenue, Miami, FL 33136.
E-mail addresses: rayner_rodriguez@yahoo.com; acaicedo@med.miami.edu

Endocrinol Metab Clin N Am 42 (2013) 39–56
http://dx.doi.org/10.1016/j.ecl.2012.11.001
0889-8529/13/$ – see front matter © 2013 Elsevier Inc. All rights reserved.

in particular of human islets, and (2) it has been difficult to discern the effects auto-nomic fibers have locally on islet cell physiology from the confounding effects the autonomic input has simultaneously on many other organs. This article gives a brief overview of the literature on islet innervation, and discusses the difficulties inherent to this research. It then focuses on approaches that are currently used to circumvent major limitations of studying the structural and functional innervation of the islet.

COMPONENTS OF THE AUTONOMIC NERVOUS SYSTEM IN ISLETS OF LANGERHANS

Based on numerous studies, the consensus is that the endocrine pancreas is richly innervated by the autonomic nervous system.[3–8] Parasympathetic and sympathetic nerves travel to the islet through the neurovascular stalk. Within the islets, the nerves follow the blood vessels and terminate within the pericapillary space, within the capillary basement membrane, or closely apposed to the endocrine cells.[9] These fibers do not form classic synapses with endocrine cells but have release sites near these islet cells. It has been proposed that neurotransmitters are released into the interstitial space to affect a group of adjacent islet cells.

The distribution and density of the different types of nerve fibers have been examined in several species. A dense sympathetic innervation, as identified by the presence of catecholamine-synthesizing enzymes, has been reported in rodents, dogs, and cats.[10–13] Studies based on the cholinesterase technique have revealed the parasympathetic innervation in the cat, rat, and rabbit.[14–18] Fibers containing neuropeptides have also been reported, but it is unclear whether these represent unique fiber populations or whether these peptides are localized in the autonomic fibers.[12] In addition, there is a network of sensory fibers containing the neuropeptides calcitonin gene–related peptide (GGRP) and substance P. Thus far, the innervation of human islets has been merely mentioned in a few studies.[19–21]

Although the work cited earlier provides convincing evidence that autonomic fibers innervate the islets, the precise organization of islet innervation is mostly unknown. Only a few markers have been used and, because these markers have not been combined in immunofluorescence studies, it is unclear how the different fiber systems relate to each other. For instance, it is not known whether the patterns of the parasympathetic and sympathetic innervations are complementary or whether they overlap in specific regions of the islet. There have been few attempts to identify peptides as cotransmitters in cholinergic and adrenergic fibers. Furthermore, relying on the cholinesterase technique may be misleading because esterases do not map exclusively to parasympathetic nerves. Other important prototypical cholinergic markers for the parasympathetic system (eg, choline acetyltransferase [ChAT], vesicular acetylcholine transporter [vAChT]) have barely been examined. There are no systematic analyses on how and where the axons terminate within the islets, and what particular cells they innervate. It is also obvious that the current view of islet innervation is based mainly on rodent studies, and that, given their unique cytoarchitecture, the situation in human islets may be different.[22–24]

NEUROTRANSMITTER RECEPTORS EXPRESSED ON THE PLASMA MEMBRANE OF ISLET CELLS

Parasympathetic axons and sympathetic axons release acetylcholine and noradrena-line, which act on cholinergic and adrenergic receptors, respectively. Activation of cholinergic muscarinic receptors stimulates insulin and glucagon secretion.[25–27] Release of Ca^{2+} from intracellular stores in response to muscarinic receptor activation is the major cause for the insulinotropic action, but the signaling underlying the enhanced glucagon secretion needs to be established. Activation of α2-adrenergic receptors inhibits glucose-induced insulin secretion via hyperpolarization of the β cell. Activation of β2-adrenergic receptors stimulates insulin and glucagon secretion. Thus, the actions of a neurotransmitter vary according to the activated receptor type. To add to this complexity, neuropeptides, which are also released from autonomic axons, including vasoactive intestinal peptide (VIP), neuropeptide Y, and, in some species, galanin, also have effects on islet cells.[5,28] Most of the in vitro studies have been conducted with rodent islets. Because the effects of neurotransmitter on islet endocrine cells may vary considerably between species, it will be important to establish the neurotransmitter receptor profiles in human islet cells, in particular because these could represent potential therapeutic targets.

PHYSIOLOGIC STUDIES ON THE EFFECTS OF THE AUTONOMIC NERVOUS SYSTEM ON ISLET FUNCTION

The overall effect of parasympathetic stimulation is an increase in insulin secretion. Several studies support the view that acetylcholine is released to stimulate insulin secretion. Exogenous treatment with acetylcholine or other muscarinic agonists stimulates insulin secretion in vivo. This effect can be blocked with the muscarinic antagonist atropine.[16,17] In vivo studies in the dog and the baboon reported that stimulation of the vagus nerve increases insulin secretion,[29–31] but this stimulation also increases the secretion of other islet hormones such as glucagon, somatostatin, and pancreatic polypeptide.[16,32,33] The net effect of sympathetic nerve stimulation seems to be a lowering of plasma insulin concentration. Exogenous treatment with catecholamines and electrical activation of sympathetic nerves inhibits insulin secretion in vivo.[34–36] α-Adrenergic receptor blockade counteracts this inhibition of insulin secretion,[35,37] suggesting noradrenaline as the mediator.

However, several other direct and indirect mechanisms could contribute to the effects of noradrenaline on insulin secretion: noradrenaline may activate β-adrenergic receptors on β cells and adrenergic receptors on α cells, which makes it difficult to interpret the results. Moreover, this effect cannot be attributed solely to the release of noradrenaline from nerve fibers close to β cells because other tissues innervated by the activated nerves are also stimulated. The sympathetic nervous system further exerts profound effects on the secretion of the other islet hormones. Splanchnic nerve stimulation and noradrenaline application increase glucagon secretion and decrease somatostatin secretion.[28,33,35–38] To our knowledge, similar studies have not been performed in human beings.

Autonomic innervation of the endocrine pancreas modulates function of the islet. It does not determine it. The islet can work without innervation (discussed later), but it needs nervous input to adapt the hormonal secretory output to changes in the internal and external environments. Thus, the autonomic input has a role in adjusting glucose homeostasis in response to food intake or stress.[5,39] In this sense, it is similar to autonomic input to the heart, where the parasympathetic and sympathetic inputs adjust the force and pace of the basic heartbeat in response to behavioral challenges. Moreover, the autonomic nervous input may not only be important for acutely modulating hormone secretion. As experiments in mice lacking neurotransmitter receptors have shown, it is also likely that the nervous input has a trophic role in maintaining a healthy population of β cells.[27]

SENSORY AXONS AND THE LINK TO DIABETES

In addition to the efferent fibers of the autonomic nervous system, the islets are also innervated by a network of sensory fibers. These fibers leave the pancreas along the sympathetic fibers within the splanchnic nerves and transmit information about noxious stimuli. Fibers containing the sensory neuropeptides GGRP and substance P have been observed in the endocrine pancreas. Vanilloid receptors are localized in sensory fibers and generally report pain information. Whether these fibers are involved in the regulation of islet hormone secretion remains to be determined. Recent articles suggest that eliminating the pancreatic sensory innervation dramatically affects autoimmune diabetes in NOD mice[40,41] and contributes to defective insulin secretion in the Zucker diabetic rat, an animal model for type 2 diabetes.[42] These studies raise the possibility that signals derived from the sensory component of the autonomic nervous system can alter insulin secretion and islet inflammation, thus indirectly affecting the development of autoimmunity and type 2 diabetes. However, it is unclear to what extent human islets are innervated by sensory fibers. Finding out which receptors are expressed on these fibers is crucial to the proposition that a similar mechanism provides a link between the nervous system and the natural history of diabetes in human beings.

ESTABLISHING THE ROLE OF AUTONOMIC INNERVATION OF THE ISLET IN GLUCOSE HOMEOSTASIS IS CHALLENGING

To establish that a tissue is innervated, investigators can (1) show that neurotransmitters are present within the efferent autonomic axon, (2) show that the neurotransmitter is released in response to stimulation of the efferent axon, and (3) show that specific receptors for the neurotransmitter are present on the postsynaptic cell. However, performing these studies in the pancreas is technically challenging. Many physiologic events under parasympathetic and sympathetic control can indirectly interfere with insulin or glucagon secretion. It has been difficult to differentiate the direct effects of autonomic terminals in the islet from the confounding effects of the autonomic nervous system elsewhere (eg, incretin secretion, activation of the adrenal medulla). Selective stimulation of islet innervation is difficult. For instance, to achieve a specific activation of the pancreas, investigators have to use electrical activation of the mixed autonomic nerves along a pancreatic artery with a concomitant blockade of the joint preganglionic cholinergic nerves.[35,36] Furthermore, if not applied locally, exogenous application of neurotransmitters can influence multiple organs and tissues and, as a result, the effects are the sum of a multitude of activities. An additional limitation is that the responses of islet cells to nerve stimulation can only be measured indirectly in the systemic circulation (eg, hormone plasma levels). It is not possible to record receptor activation directly in the postsynaptic cells.

As a result, although several studies suggest the involvement of the autonomic nervous system, the importance of islet innervation in regulating islet hormone secretion is unclear. The list of neurotransmitters that may modulate islet function is long and confusing because of species differences and uncertainty about the physiologic relevance of the effects observed with in vivo models. In human subjects, decreased glucose tolerance after vagotomy has been reported,[43,44] but patients who have undergone pancreas transplantation (and thus may have denervated islets) remain euglycemic without therapy.[45–48] For similar reasons, doubts exist about whether sympathetic nerve fibers exert a major influence on the basal and postprandial insulin secretory responses. The contribution of autonomic signals to the glucagon secretory response in vivo is also unclear. Autonomic activation most likely has a major role in dogs[49] and in monkeys,[50] but combined adrenergic and muscarinic cholinergic blockade has no effect on the glucagon response to hypoglycemia in humans.[51,52] Furthermore, this glucagon response is not reduced in adrenalectomized, spinal cord–sectioned, or vagotomized humans.[53–57]

We agree with other investigators[5,28] that the lack of experimental tools has prevented critical demonstrations of the effects of autonomic innervation. A successful new approach has been to generate mutant mice lacking a particular neurotransmitter receptor in a particular islet cell. Thus, studies of knockout mice lacking the M3 muscarinic receptor in β cells showed that M3 receptors have an important role in promoting insulin secretion and maintaining glucose homeostasis.[27] This strategy eliminates potential confounding factors caused by the widespread distribution of autonomic neurotransmitter receptors. However, this approach is too cumbersome to allow a larger screening of the role of the many putative receptors on islet cells and it cannot be used to examine the physiologic role of islet cell receptors in humans. Furthermore, these receptors are not used exclusively to mediate neural input and could be responding to humoral and paracrine signals.

NEW APPROACHES TO STUDYING THE ANATOMIC ASPECTS OF ISLET INNERVATION

A major hurdle to studying innervation patterns is related to the structure of the neuronal axon. Histologic examination of axons is difficult because they are elongated, meandering, and thin structures. Although an axon can be longer than a meter, it is generally less than 5 μm thick. Axons are bundled in nerves, but when they reach their target tissues they branch extensively and run in complex pathways through the tissue parenchyma, often along blood vessels, to establish contacts with effector cells. On their way to their final target, axons may contact many different types of cells and traverse tissues with a variety of functions. Autonomic axons, in particular, do not form specialized terminal endings but secrete their neurotransmitter content at axonal varicosities in the close vicinity of target cells. The lack of a well-defined terminal structure makes it difficult to determine whether or not a particular cell type is innervated by the autonomic nervous system.

In view of these difficulties, how can the innervation of the pancreatic islet be studied? To visualize axons, investigators can use axonal tracing techniques in animal models.[58] With retrograde and anterograde axonal tracing, the origin of the innervation as well as the terminal innervation patterns can be determined in detail. These experiments cannot be performed in human beings. Instead, investigators most commonly detect molecules that serve as axonal markers. These molecules can be targeted with specific antibodies using immunohistochemical techniques. The markers include both structural (ie, neurofilaments, myelin, acetylated actin) and functional molecules such as neurotransmitters and proteins involved in synthesis, packaging, secretion, or degradation of neurotransmitters (ie, biosynthetic enzymes, vesicular transporters). Labeled axons are then visualized using bright field or fluorescence microscopy (**Fig. 1**). In most studies, data are presented as micrographs showing labeled axonal shafts and varicosities within the tissue of interest. Because these images are generally taken from thin sections (5–15 μm), only fragments of the axons or dispersed varicosities are visualized. Often, these cannot be discerned as neuronal elements or even be distinguished from staining artifacts. In addition, the results are qualitative because only a few images can be shown in an article. As a consequence, many results in the literature can be considered anecdotal.

To be able to understand the innervation pattern of an organ it is crucial to visualize large portions of the axonal plexus penetrating the tissue. This visualization can be accomplished by using the immunostaining approaches mentioned earlier on thicker histologic sections (40–60 μm). Labeled axons are then imaged with confocal microscopy to produce Z-stacks of confocal images. These Z-stacks are used to render the axonal plexus in 3 dimensions. In these three-dimensional reconstructions, axon

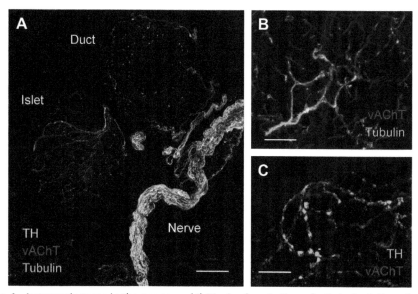

Fig. 1. Autonomic axons in the pancreas. (*A*) Maximal projection of a Z-stack of 40 confocal images (Z step 0.5 μm) of a mouse pancreatic section showing axons labeled for acetylated tubulin (*green*), vAChT (*red*), and tyrosine hydroxylase (TH, *light blue*). Note that acetylated tubulin is present in the entire axon whereas vAChT and TH are restricted to axon varicosities. TH and vAChT label noradrenergic sympathetic and cholinergic parasympathetic axons, respectively. (*B*) At higher magnification, tubulin-stained axons are beaded with vAChT-positive varicosities. (*C*) Sympathetic and parasympathetic axons run together in the same nerve tracts, as shown by the close association between TH-labeled and vAChT-labeled axons. Scale bars 20 μm (*A*) And 10 μm (*B, C*).

trajectories and branching can be followed, and the terminal fields of axons become visible as agglomerations of varicosities. When the cells of the innervated tissue are labeled with cell-specific markers, it is possible to determine which cell populations are within the terminal field of an axon, and this gives a first hint of which cells are targeted by the nervous input. However, most studies of islet innervation have not attempted to identify the cellular targets of innervation. As a consequence, in many published images, axons seem lost in the pancreatic parenchyma in search for a target.

How can the cells that are targets of autonomic axons in the islet be determined? This is not straightforward because autonomic axons do not show the same terminal specializations that are typical of axonal endings in the central nervous system or at neuromuscular endplates. To help address this issue, 2 assumptions can be made: (1) varicosities are the sites at which neurotransmitters are released, and cells closely apposed to these varicosities can be considered targets[59]; and (2) because of the limits of optical resolution, close apposition between axonal varicosities and target cells (<200 nm) can be revealed as an overlap in the axonal and the cellular labeling. These assumptions not only define autonomic innervation conceptually but also provide a strategy to visualize the contacts established with effector cells. Using this approach, we recently determined the cellular targets for parasympathetic and sympathetic axons in mouse and human islets.[60] We dissected out in detail the preferential axonal targets in the islet and, based on these anatomic data, proposed that the autonomic nervous system uses different mechanisms to regulate islet function in mouse and human islets.

It is likely that the anatomic observations have a functional correlate, but, to be accurate and predictive, this extrapolation requires in-depth structural studies and should include quantitative results. However, few studies have provided numbers on islet innervation, mostly because the technology to measure axonal volumes in the tissue or contacts with target cells was not available until recently. With modern software applications, it is now possible to determine the volume of labeled structures within a defined tissue volume. The fraction of axonal volume to tissue volume gives an estimate of innervation densities that can be used to examine differences between tissues, species, or experimental conditions. For instance, the innervation density in the endocrine pancreas can be compared with that in the exocrine pancreas, which reveals a stronger innervation of the islet in the mouse pancreas.[60] The volume of the overlap between the axonal staining and target cell staining can similarly be used to determine whether a cell population is innervated. Using this approach, we found that vascular cells, but not endocrine cells, are the major targets of sympathetic innervation in the human islet.[60]

These examples show that it is feasible to get quantitative estimates of innervation patterns, without which studies are only subjective or anecdotal. There is a series of technical difficulties and critical checkpoints to be considered when visualizing pancreatic innervation, in particular in human specimens:

1. Well-preserved human tissue specimens are not always available because pancreatic tissue is sensitive to postmortem damage. Specimens come from cadaveric donors and the endocrine tissue is surrounded by acinar tissue loaded with digestive enzymes. Many specimens may be needed to get satisfactory results.
2. Effective and fast fixation of the pancreatic tissue and the right choice of the fixative agent is needed to preserve the marker epitopes on target molecules, which will help detect axonal markers. For instance, long fixation in formalin, the default fixative agent used in most pathology laboratories, may impair antigenicity. It is important to perform control experiments to establish that antigenicity is not lost and that antibodies are recognizing the target proteins. The exocrine pancreas surrounding the islets can be inspected for the presence of labeled axons in major nerves or running along major blood vessels (**Fig. 2**). In principle, staining of these axons should be conserved across species.
3. Inclusion or embedding of the tissue and the process of deembedding (ie, deparaffinization) may impair antigenicity. We recommend sectioning the fixed, frozen, optimal cutting temperature (OCT)–embedded pancreas on a cryostat microtome.
4. In general, tissues are cut into sections of cellular or subcellular thickness (5–15 μm), which is not suitable for visualization of thin and elongated structural elements. In these thin sections, it is difficult to distinguish between transected fibers, varicosities, and staining artifacts. Thicker sections (40–60 μm) are preferable.
5. Staining procedures, including the best use of detergents and optimized incubation times, are crucial to allow optimal penetration of antibodies. Antigen retrieval or amplification of the immunostaining staining may be necessary to visualize axonal markers.
6. Choice of commercial antibodies recognizing axon-specific markers is pivotal (**Table 1**). Using several antibodies for each axonal marker may be needed.
7. A state-of-the-art confocal microscope to acquire images with the optimal resolution (60× objective lenses with high numerical aperture) is required to image thin axons and small varicosities. Z-stacks of confocal images have to be acquired at the optimal z resolution to allow three-dimensional rendering of images.

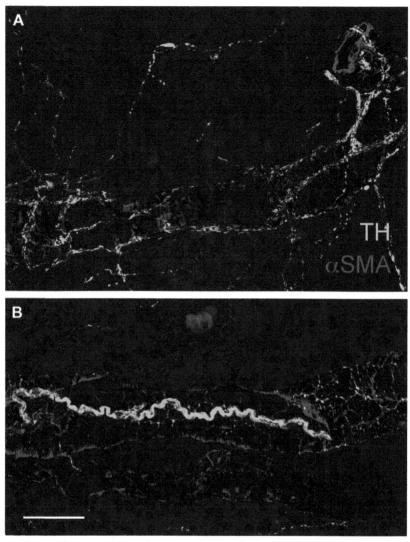

Fig. 2. Control immunostaining in the pancreas. Maximal projection of a Z-stack of 40 confocal images (Z step 0.5 μm) of a human (*A*) and a mouse (*B*) pancreatic section showing vascular smooth muscle cells of a large artery labeled for α smooth muscle actin (aSMA, *red*) and the sympathetic nerves running along the vessel labeled for TH (*green*). Note that the staining patterns are similar in both species. Scale bar 20 μm.

8. Cellular imaging software (eg, Volocity 3D Image Analysis Software, PerkinElmer) is necessary to reconstruct axonal tress and reveal clusters of varicosities in 3 dimensions (**Fig. 3**). Software is also needed to measure the volumes of labeled structures and to detect cell contacts as defined by staining overlap.

9. Once volumes of labeled structures are measured, the axonal density per tissue volume can be calculated. The density of contacts of axons with specific types of cells can also be calculated as the ratio of the volume of the staining overlap to the volume of the staining of the cell population of interest. It is important to

select adequate detection parameters to filter out background noise and staining artifacts (eg, by carefully selecting detection thresholds). A limitation of this approach is that axon shafts close to target cells may also be included in the analyses. To avoid this, it is preferable to use axon markers that are concentrated in varicosities (eg, vesicular neurotransmitter transporters).

PHYSIOLOGIC APPROACHES TO STUDYING INNERVATION

In vivo investigation of the influence of innervation on islet function has mostly been limited to studies in which the effects of systemic intervention (ie, stimulation of the vagus nerve, exogenous application of neurotransmitters) are measured with systemic metabolic readouts (ie, blood insulin levels). Under these circumstances, the stimulation is not specific to the islet, which raises a series of issues. First, the parasympathetic and sympathetic branches of the autonomic nervous system control many physiologic events in the body. Application of agonists or antagonists and stimulation or transection of the autonomic nerves can indirectly affect islet hormone secretion. Second, autonomic axons release a panoply of neurotransmitters and neuropeptides, which makes it difficult to interpret the effects of autonomic input on islet hormone secretion in vivo. For instance, vagal stimulation can release at least 5 neurotransmitters (acetylcholine, VIP, pituitary adenylate cyclase activating polypeptide, gastrin-releasing peptide, and nitric oxide), the relative contribution of which differs between organs and species. Third, several intestinal hormones, particularly glucose-dependent insulin-releasing peptide (GIP) and glucagonlike peptide-1 (GLP-1), potently increase insulin secretion. GIP-secreting cells and GLP-1-secreting cells express neurotransmitter receptors, and both the stimulation of autonomic nerves and agonists stimulate their release. Fourth, stimulation of autonomic input can change regional blood flow, which may affect islet hormone secretion into the bloodstream. Selective stimulation of pancreas innervation is difficult,[35,36] and specific stimulation of axons contacting cells within the islet may never be achieved in vivo, in particular in the human pancreas. For these reasons, results need to be interpreted with caution.

Even if it were possible to selectively stimulate islet innervation, it would only be possible to measure the effects on islet cells indirectly, namely by using changes in hormone blood concentration as a readout. However, hormone levels in the blood are the end product of a chain of events occurring in the islet as well as downstream after interactions with target tissues. The autonomic nervous input may directly influence the secretion of islet hormones, which may act as paracrine signals regulating the secretion of other islet hormones, or sympathetic input to islet blood vessels may change regional blood flow and increase hormone release into the circulation. The current readouts do not allow the proximal mechanisms used by the local innervation to regulate islet function to be discerned. A common approach to detecting parasympathetic activation of islet function is to measure the concentration of pancreatic polypeptide (PP) in the circulation, because PP is released in response to vagal activation.[8] Although it is an important tool for measuring vagal activity in the pancreas, a caveat here is that PP blood levels may not reflect parasympathetic input to most islets because endocrine cells producing and releasing PP are concentrated in a distinct region of the human pancreas in islets almost devoid of β and α cells.[61–63]

New, creative approaches are needed to overcome the limitations of studying the functional role of islet innervation. Emerging efforts include in vivo studies in human beings using pharmacologic agents that act selectively on neurotransmitter release from autonomic axons. Thus, endogenous release of noradrenaline can be specifically

Table 1
List of antibodies used and immunostaining patterns in the pancreas

| Antibody to | Host | Company | Catalog No. | Reactivity to Human | | | Reactivity to Mouse | | |
| | | | | Axons | | | Axons | | |
				Varicosities	Shaft	Others	Varicosities	Shaft	Others
Synapsin I/II	Rabbit	SySy	106002	+++	+++		+++	+++	Neuroinsular complex
	Mouse Mab	SySy	106011C5	+++	+++		+++	+++	Neuroinsular complex
	Guinea Pig	SySy	106004	+	+		+	+	–
Tyroxine hydroxylase	Rabbit	Chemicon	AB152	+++	+++	β Cell subset[a]	+++	+++	β cell subset
	Sheep	Chemicon	AB1542	+++	+++	β Cell subset[a]	+++	+++	β Cell subset
	Mouse MAb	Sigma	T1299	–	–	–	–	–	–
	Chicken	Chemicon	AB9702	++	++	β Cell subset[a]	++	++	β Cell subset
Vesicular acetylcholine transporter	Rabbit	SySy	139103	+++	+	α Cells	+++	+	Neuroinsular complex
	Rabbit	Sigma	V5387	+	+	α Cells	+	+	Neuroinsular complex
	Goat	BD-Pharmigen	556337	–	–	–	–	–	–
	Mouse MAb	Phoenix Pharmaceuticals	H-V005	–	–	–	–	–	–
Choline acetyl transferase	Goat	Chemicon	AB144P	++	+	α Cells[b]	++	+	Neuroinsular complex[b]
	Rabbit	Chemicon	AB143	+	+	–	+	+	–
	Rabbit	Pierce	OSC00008W	–	–	–	–	–	–
Choline transporter	Rabbit	Chemicon	AB5966	–	–	–	–	–	–
Vesicular monoamine transporter 2	Rabbit	SySy	138302	++	++	–	++	++	β Cell subset
	Rabbit	Phoenix Pharmaceuticals	H-V004	–	–	–	–	–	–

Antigen	Species	Company	Catalog no.	Staining 1	Staining 2	Staining 3
Dopamine β hydroxilase	Sheep	Abcam	Ab19353	–	–	–
Neuron-specific enolase	Chicken	Chemicon	AB9698	–	–	– Endocrine cells
	Mouse MAb	Chemicon	MAB324	–	–	–
Protein gene product 9.5	Rabbit	AbD Serotec	7863–0507	+	+++ Endocrine cell nuclei	+++ Endocrine cell nuclei, neuroinsular complex
Acetylated α-tubulin	Mouse MAb	Sigma	T6793	+	+++ Primary cilia, endocrine cells	+++ Primary cilia, neuroinsular complex
β-Tubulin (TuJ)	Rabbit	Covance	MRB4358	–	–	+++ Neuroinsular complex
S100B	Rabbit	Abcam	ab14688	–	–	–
Neurofilament H	Chicken	Neuromics	CH22104	++	++	++ Neuroinsular complex
Neurofilament 200	Rabbit	Sigma	N4142	+	+	+
α-NG2 condroitin sulfate proteoglycan	Rabbit	Chemicon	AB5320	–	– Pericytes in islet	–
Human CD-31 (PECAM)	Mouse MAb	BD-Pharmigen	550389	–	– Endothelial cells	– Endothelial cells
Actin α-smooth muscle	Mouse MAb	Sigma	C6198	–	– Smooth muscle cells	– Smooth muscle cells
Cytokeratin-19	Mouse MAb	Bio-Genex	AM246-5M	–	– Ductal cells	– Ductal cells
Insulin	Guinea Pig	Dako	A0564	–	– β Cells	– β Cells
Glucagon	Mouse MAb	Sigma	G2654-5	–	– α Cells	– α Cells
Somatostatin	Rat Mab	Chemicon	MAB354	–	– δ Cells	– δ Cells

Abbreviation: PECAM, platelet endothelial cell adhesion molecule.
a In 1 out of 10 examined human pancreas samples.
b Cell staining obtained with tyramide signal amplification.

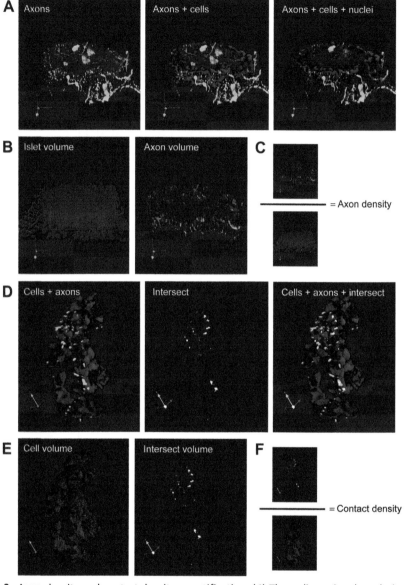

Fig. 3. Axon density and contact density quantification. (*A*) Three-dimensional rendering of a Z-stack of confocal images (n = 40) of a mouse pancreatic section stained for TH (*green*), glucagon (*red*), and diamidino phenylindole (DAPI) (*blue*). (*B*) Islet volume (in voxels) is determined by outlining the islet using DAPI staining. The volume of axonal staining is determined within this islet volume. (*C*) The axon (innervation) density is calculated as the quotient axon volume/islet volume. (*D*) TH-labeled axons can be seen in close proximity to glucagon-labeled α cells. Shown is a higher magnification and rotated image of the islet in (*A*). The proximity of axons to target cells can be detected using an algorithm in Volocity software (intersect). Intersect between axons and cells is shown in yellow. Note that few axonal varicosities contact target cells (*yellow* and *green* overlap in the merged image on the right). (*E*) Cellular (cell) volume is determined based on cell immunostaining, and intersect volume is determined as the close proximity or overlap of axon and cell immunostaining. (*F*) The contact density is calculated as the quotient intersect volume/cellular volume. *Adapted from* Rodriguez-Diaz R, Abdulreda MH, Formoso AL, et al. Innervation patterns of autonomic axons in the human endocrine pancreas. Cell Metab 2011;14:45–54; with permission.

stimulated from sympathetic axons by infusing the indirect sympathomimetic agent tyramine.[64] This treatment produces only modest effects on potentially confounding circulating noradrenaline levels. Using this approach, an effect of sympathetic innervation on insulin secretion was eventually shown in human beings.[64] Whether this effect was mediated by axons acting directly on β cells or by other mechanisms in the islet could not be shown. However, monitoring islet activity in the organism is challenging, and noninvasive or minimally invasive technologies to monitor islet cell function with sufficient spatial resolution have not been developed.

To study β cell function in an intact environment, organotypic pancreatic slices containing islets are used for electrophysiologic recordings.[65–67] This preparation preserves intraislet cellular communication and islet architecture in their native states, including the distal portion of the autonomic innervation. In principle, it should be feasible to stimulate local axons electrically while recording cellular responses in the islet, which would allow the characterization of the local mechanisms by which axons influence endocrine cell function. This approach has not been extended to the human pancreas, but it should be possible to produce living pancreatic slices from human pancreatic biopsies. Of course, in this preparation the pancreas is isolated from the organism and therefore these ex vivo experiments cannot determine the effects that the islet's nervous input has on glucose homeostasis.

Studying the influence of innervation on islet function in vivo in the pancreas of human beings may not be feasible. Recent efforts to image β cells in vivo include magnetic resonance imaging and position emission tomography.[68,69] Such methods likely will improve the quantification of transplanted islet mass but have low spatial resolution and do not allow functional monitoring of islets. An alternative strategy is to make human islets accessible for imaging by transplanting them into an animal model. Islets have been imaged after transplantation under the kidney capsule, where it has been possible to visualize the revascularization process.[70,71] However, the instability and inaccessibility of this transplantation site makes this approach challenging, in particular for functional or longitudinal studies.

To dissociate the neural effects from hormonal and other confounding effects and to record islet function locally and systemically after manipulation of the neural input, investigators could use an experimental platform in which islets are transplanted into the anterior chamber of the eye for functional monitoring.[72–74] In the early 1870s, van Dooremaal[75] made the observation that tumor cells injected into the anterior chamber of the eye formed progressively growing tumors. Since then, the anterior chamber of the eye has been widely used as a model system to study the biology of several tissues. Ovaries have been transplanted into the anterior eye chamber to study the physiology of ovulation,[76,77] and a wide variety of peripheral and central nervous tissues have been shown to proliferate and mature histologically after intraocular transplantation.[78,79] This site has also been used extensively to study the survival and growth of pancreatic tissue grafts.[80,81] Human xenografts survive in the anterior chamber of the eye of athymic nude rodents, where they become strongly and appropriately innervated.[79,82–84]

In this transplantation site, biologic phenomena can be monitored repeatedly without invasive procedures because the cornea is transparent. The grafts are easily vascularized and innervated because of the rich blood and nerve supply of the iris that forms the bed of the anterior chamber of the eye. The iris contains noradrenergic and cholinergic nerve fibers that control pupillary diameter. These fibers have been shown to innervate the intraocular grafts appropriately and can be specifically activated by changing the illumination[78,85] or by topical drug application. Therefore, the autonomic input to the grafted tissue can be modulated noninvasively and locally. Taking advantage of these features can provide an experimental platform that allows local, specific manipulation of the neural input to the islets while imaging islet cell function in real time in response to neural activation. To measure the effects of this manipulation on glucose homeostasis, systemic readouts such as detection of glucose and hormone plasma levels during glucose and insulin tolerance tests can be used. Local, cellular readouts include imaging of cytoplasmic $[Ca^{2+}]$, electrophysiologic recordings, or measurements of blood flow.

A potential limitation is that human tissue is not innervated to the same degree as mouse tissue because of species incompatibilities. However, these species incompatibilities may not be problematic because human tissues have been successfully transplanted into the mouse eye, where they become strongly and appropriately innervated.[79,83,84] It is also important to clarify that the intraocular islet grafts are not under the control of the autonomous nervous system as they are in the pancreas. Thus, it is not possible to study the influences of feeding behavior and stress on nervous input to the islet. However, it can be advantageous that islets are disconnected from this circuit and still work appropriately. Cutting islet grafts from their natural nervous connections and replacing them with an artificial innervation may be the only way to distinguish the direct effects of parasympathetic and sympathetic innervation from all other confounding factors that can affect islet function and survival. Autonomic axons in islet grafts in the eye can be activated selectively and noninvasively, enabling acute and chronic intervention while the physiologic effects of islet innervation are monitored in a living organism.

CONCLUDING REMARKS

There is a gap in the knowledge about how the nervous system controls human glucose homeostasis, and there are few comprehensive morphologic studies of the innervation of the human islet of Langerhans. Malfunction of the islet of Langerhans is a hallmark of diabetes, a condition affecting millions. Despite many years of investigation, a clear picture of human islet microanatomy is slowly emerging. A consolidated structural model that puts together the different subsets of human endocrine cells with vascular, immune, and neural elements is still missing. To understand the biology of the islet also requires establishing functional links between these different structures in vivo. A cohesive picture of the microanatomy of the islet of Langerhans will help identify the sequential events leading to the failure of this microorgan during diabetes.

REFERENCES

1. Bernard C. Leçons De Physiologie Expérimentale Appliquée À La Médecine. Paris: Bailliere; 1855.
2. Langerhans P, Morrison H. Contributions to the microscopic anatomy of the pancreas. Baltimore (MD): The Johns Hopkins Press; 1937.
3. Woods S, Porte DJ. Neural control of the endocrine pancreas. Physiol Rev 1974; 54:596–619.
4. Satin L, Kinard T. Neurotransmitters and their receptors in the islets of Langerhans of the pancreas: what messages do acetylcholine, glutamate, and GABA transmit? Endocrine 1998;8:213–23.
5. Ahrén B. Autonomic regulation of islet hormone secretion–implications for health and disease. Diabetologia 2000;43:393–410.
6. Gilon P, Henquin J. Mechanisms and physiological significance of the cholinergic control of pancreatic beta-cell function. Endocr Rev 2001;22:565–604.

7. Gerald J, Taborsky J. Handbook of physiology. New York: Oxford University Press, American Physiological Society; 2001.

8. Teff KL. How neural mediation of anticipatory and compensatory insulin release helps us tolerate food. Physiol Behav 2011;103:44–50.

9. Bonner-Weir S. Islets of Langerhans: morphology and postnatal growth. Boston: Lippincott Williams & Wilkins; 2005.

10. Cegrell L. Catecholamines in pancreas of human fetuses. Acta Physiol Scand 1968;73(S314):14–6.

11. Ahrén B, Ericson L, Lundquist I, et al. Adrenergic innervation of pancreatic islets and modulation of insulin secretion by the sympatho-adrenal system. Cell Tissue Res 1981;216:15–30.

12. Ahrén B, Böttcher G, Kowalyk S, et al. Galanin is co-localized with noradrenaline and neuropeptide Y in dog pancreas and celiac ganglion. Cell Tissue Res 1990; 261:49–58.

13. Stach W, Radke R. Innervation of islands of Langerhans. Light and electron microscopic studies of the pancreas in laboratory animals. Endokrinologie 1982;79:210–20 [in German].

14. Coupland R. The innervation of pancreas of the rat, cat and rabbit as revealed by the cholinesterase technique. J Anat 1958;92:143–9.

15. Esterhuizen A, Spriggs T, Lever J. Nature of islet-cell innervation in the cat pancreas. Diabetes 1968;17:33–6.

16. Ahrén B, Taborsky GJ, Porte D. Neuropeptidergic versus cholinergic and adrenergic regulation of islet hormone secretion. Diabetologia 1986;29:827–36.

17. Brunicardi F, Shavelle D, Andersen D. Neural regulation of the endocrine pancreas. Int J Pancreatol 1995;18:177–95.

18. Love J, Szebeni K. Morphology and histochemistry of the rabbit pancreatic innervation. Pancreas 1999;18:53–64.

19. Ahrén B, Berggren PO, Rorsman P, et al. Neuropeptides in the regulation of islet hormone secretion–localization, effects and mode of action. Adv Exp Med Biol 1991;291:129–42.

20. Shimosegawa T, Asakura T, Kashimura J, et al. Neurons containing gastrin releasing peptide-like immunoreactivity in the human pancreas. Pancreas 1993; 8:403–12.

21. Ding WG, Kimura H, Fujimura M, et al. Neuropeptide Y and peptide YY immunoreactivities in the pancreas of various vertebrates. Peptides 1997;18:1523–9.

22. Brissova M, Fowler M, Nicholson W, et al. Assessment of human pancreatic islet architecture and composition by laser scanning confocal microscopy. J Histochem Cytochem 2005;53:1087–97.

23. Cabrera O, Berman D, Kenyon N, et al. The unique cytoarchitecture of human pancreatic islets has implications for islet cell function. Proc Natl Acad Sci U S A 2006;103:2334–9.

24. Bosco D, Armanet M, Morel P, et al. Unique arrangement of alpha- and beta-cells in human islets of Langerhans. Diabetes 2010;59:1202–10.

25. Verspohl EJ, Tacke R, Mutschler E, et al. Muscarinic receptor subtypes in rat pancreatic islets: binding and functional studies. Eur J Pharmacol 1990;178:303–11.

26. Havel P, Akpan J, Curry D, et al. Autonomic control of pancreatic polypeptide and glucagon secretion during neuroglucopenia and hypoglycemia in mice. Am J Physiol 1993;265:R246–54.

27. Gautam D, Han S, Hamdan F, et al. A critical role for beta cell M3 muscarinic acetylcholine receptors in regulating insulin release and blood glucose homeostasis in vivo. Cell Metab 2006;3:449–61.

28. Dunning BE, Taborsky GJ. Galanin–sympathetic neurotransmitter in endocrine pancreas? Diabetes 1988;37:1157–62.

29. Daniel PM, Henderson JR. The effect of vagal stimulation on plasma insulin and glucose levels in the baboon. J Physiol 1967;192:317–27.

30. Frohman LA, Ezdinli EZ, Javid R. Effect of vagotomy and vagal stimulation on insulin secretion. Diabetes 1967;16:443–8.

31. Kaneto A, Kosaka K, Nakao K. Effects of stimulation of the vagus nerve on insulin secretion. Endocrinology 1967;80:530–6.

32. Alejandro R, Feldman E, Bloom A, et al. Effects of cyclosporin on insulin and C-peptide secretion in healthy beagles. Diabetes 1989;38:698–703.

33. Holst JJ, Grønholt R, Schaffalitzky de Muckadell OB, et al. Nervous control of pancreatic endocrine secretion in pigs. I. Insulin and glucagon responses to electrical stimulation of the vagus nerves. Acta Physiol Scand 1981;111:1–7.

34. Porte D, Williams RH. Inhibition of insulin release by norepinephrine in man. Science 1966;152:1248–50.

35. Bloom SR, Edwards AV. Characteristics of the neuroendocrine responses to stimulation of the splanchnic nerves in bursts in the conscious calf. J Physiol 1984; 346:533–45.

36. Ahrén B, Veith RC, Taborsky GJ. Sympathetic nerve stimulation versus pancreatic norepinephrine infusion in the dog: (1). Effects on basal release of insulin and glucagon. Endocrinology 1987;121:323–31.

37. Kurose T, Seino Y, Nishi S, et al. Mechanism of sympathetic neural regulation of insulin, somatostatin, and glucagon secretion. Am J Physiol 1990;258:E220–7.

38. Holst JJ, Jensen SL, Knuhtsen S, et al. Autonomic nervous control of pancreatic somatostatin secretion. Am J Physiol 1983;245:E542–8.

39. Havel PJ, Taborsky GJ. The contribution of the autonomic nervous system to changes of glucagon and insulin secretion during hypoglycemic stress. Endocr Rev 1989;10:332–50.

40. Winer S, Tsui H, Lau A, et al. Autoimmune islet destruction in spontaneous type 1 diabetes is not beta-cell exclusive. Nat Med 2003;9:198–205.

41. Razavi R, Chan Y, Afifiyan FN, et al. TRPV1+ sensory neurons control beta cell stress and islet inflammation in autoimmune diabetes. Cell 2006;127: 1123–35.

42. Gram D, Ahrén B, Nagy I, et al. Capsaicin-sensitive sensory fibers in the islets of Langerhans contribute to defective insulin secretion in Zucker diabetic rat, an animal model for some aspects of human type 2 diabetes. Eur J Neurosci 2007; 25:213–23.

43. Linquette M, Fourlinnie JC, Lagache G. Study of blood sugar and insulin after vagotomy and pyloroplasty in man. Ann Endocrinol (Paris) 1969;30:96–102 [in French].

44. Hakanson R, Liedberg G, Lundquist I. Effect of vagal denervation on insulin release after oral and intravenous glucose. Experientia 1971;27:460–1.

45. Pozza G, Bosi E, Secchi A, et al. Metabolic control of type I (insulin dependent) diabetes after pancreas transplantation. Br Med J (Clin Res Ed) 1985;291: 510–3.

46. Diem P, Redmon J, Abid M, et al. Glucagon, catecholamine and pancreatic polypeptide secretion in type I diabetic recipients of pancreas allografts. J Clin Invest 1990;86:2008–13.

47. Blackman J, Polonsky K, Jaspan J, et al. Insulin secretory profiles and C-peptide clearance kinetics at 6 months and 2 years after kidney-pancreas transplantation. Diabetes 1992;41:1346–54.

48. Madsbad S, Christiansen E, Tibell A, et al. Beta-cell dysfunction following successful segmental pancreas transplantation. Danish-Swedish Study Group of Metabolic Effect of Pancreas Transplantation. Transplant Proc 1994;26:469–70.

49. Havel P, Taborsky G. The autonomic nervous system and insulin secretion. London: Smith Gordon; 1994. p. 343–51.

50. Havel PJ, Valverde C. Autonomic mediation of glucagon secretion during insulin-induced hypoglycemia in rhesus monkeys. Diabetes 1996;45:960–6.

51. Hilsted J, Frandsen H, Holst JJ, et al. Plasma glucagon and glucose recovery after hypoglycemia: the effect of total autonomic blockade. Acta Endocrinol (Copenh) 1991;125:466–9.

52. Towler DA, Havlin CE, Craft S, et al. Mechanism of awareness of hypoglycemia. Perception of neurogenic (predominantly cholinergic) rather than neuroglycopenic symptoms. Diabetes 1993;42:1791–8.

53. Ensinck JW, Walter RM, Palmer JP, et al. Glucagon responses to hypoglycemia in adrenalectomized man. Metabolism 1976;25:227–32.

54. Brodows RG, Campbell RG, Al-Aziz AJ. Lack of central autonomic regulation of substrate during early fasting in man. Metabolism 1976;25:803–7.

55. Palmer JP, Henry DP, Benson JW, et al. Glucagon response to hypoglycemia in sympathectomized man. J Clin Invest 1976;57:522–5.

56. Palmer JP, Werner PL, Hollander P, et al. Evaluation of the control of glucagon secretion by the parasympathetic nervous system in man. Metabolism 1979;28:549–52.

57. Corral R, Frier B. Acute hypoglycemia in man: neural control of pancreatic islet cell function. Metabolism 1981;30:160–4.

58. Caicedo A, Herbert H. Topography of descending projections from the inferior colliculus to auditory brainstem nuclei in the rat. J Comp Neurol 1993;328:377–92.

59. Burnstock G. Autonomic neurotransmission: 60 years since Sir Henry Dale. Annu Rev Pharmacol Toxicol 2009;49:1–30.

60. Rodriguez-Diaz R, Abdulreda MH, Formoso AL, et al. Innervation patterns of autonomic axons in the human endocrine pancreas. Cell Metab 2011;14:45–54.

61. Rahier J, Goebbels R, Henquin J. Cellular composition of the human diabetic pancreas. Diabetologia 1983;24:366–71.

62. Orci L, Malaisse-Lagae F, Baetens D, et al. Pancreatic-polypeptide-rich regions in human pancreas. Lancet 1978;2:1200–1.

63. Baetens D, Malaisse-Lagae F, Perrelet A, et al. Endocrine pancreas: three-dimensional reconstruction shows two types of islets of Langerhans. Science 1979;206:1323–5.

64. Gilliam LK, Palmer JP, Taborsky GJ. Tyramine-mediated activation of sympathetic nerves inhibits insulin secretion in humans. J Clin Endocrinol Metab 2007;92:4035–8.

65. Speier S, Rupnik M. A novel approach to in situ characterization of pancreatic beta-cells. Pflugers Arch 2003;446:553–8.

66. Meneghel-Rozzo T, Rozzo A, Poppi L, et al. In vivo and in vitro development of mouse pancreatic beta-cells in organotypic slices. Cell Tissue Res 2004;316:295–303.

67. Huang YC, Rupnik M, Gaisano HY. Unperturbed islet α-cell function examined in mouse pancreas tissue slices. J Physiol 2011;589:395–408.

68. Arifin DR, Bulte JW. Imaging of pancreatic islet cells. Diabetes Metab Res Rev 2011;27:761–6.

69. Malaisse WJ, Maedler K. Imaging of the β-cells of the islets of Langerhans. Diabetes Res Clin Pract 2012;98(1):11–8.

70. Bertera S, Geng X, Tawadrous Z, et al. Body window-enabled in vivo multicolor imaging of transplanted mouse islets expressing an insulin-timer fusion protein. Biotechniques 2003;35:718–22.
71. Nyqvist D, Köhler M, Wahlstedt H, et al. Donor islet endothelial cells participate in formation of functional vessels within pancreatic islet grafts. Diabetes 2005;54:2287–93.
72. Speier S, Nyqvist D, Kohler M, et al. Noninvasive high-resolution in vivo imaging of cell biology in the anterior chamber of the mouse eye. Nat Protoc 2008;3:1278–86.
73. Speier S, Nyqvist D, Cabrera O, et al. Noninvasive in vivo imaging of pancreatic islet cell biology. Nat Med 2008;14:574–8.
74. Perez VL, Caicedo A, Berman DM, et al. The anterior chamber of the eye as a clinical transplantation site for the treatment of diabetes: a study in a baboon model of diabetes. Diabetologia 2011;54:1121–6.
75. Dooremaal V. Die Entwicklung der in fremden Grund versetzten lebenden Geweba Albrecht Von Graefes. Arch Ophthalmol 1873;19:358–73.
76. Goodman L. Observations on transplanted immature ovaries in the eye of the adult male and female rats. Anat Rec 1934;59:223–51.
77. Falck B. Site of production of oestrogen in rat ovary as studied in micro-transplants. Acta Physiol Scand Suppl 1959;47:1–101.
78. Taylor D, Seiger A, Freedman R, et al. Electrophysiological analysis reinnervation of transplants in the anterior chamber of the eye by the autonomic ground plexus of the iris. Proc Natl Acad Sci U S A 1978;75:1009–12.
79. Bickford-Wimer P, Granholm AC, Bygdeman M, et al. Human fetal cerebellar and cortical tissue transplanted to the anterior eye chamber of athymic rats: electrophysiological and structural studies. Proc Natl Acad Sci U S A 1987;84:5957–61.
80. Adeghate E, Donáth T. Morphological findings in long-term pancreatic tissue transplants in the anterior eye chamber of rats. Pancreas 1990;5:298–305.
81. Adeghate E, Donáth T. Transplantation of tissue grafts into the anterior eye chamber: a method to study intrinsic neurons. Brain Res Brain Res Protoc 2000;6:33–9.
82. Olson L, Strömberg I, Bygdeman M, et al. Human fetal tissues grafted to rodent hosts: structural and functional observations of brain, adrenal and heart tissues in oculo. Exp Brain Res 1987;67:163–78.
83. Granholm AC, Eriksdotter-Nilsson M, Strömberg I, et al. Morphological and electrophysiological studies of human hippocampal transplants in the anterior eye chamber of athymic nude rats. Exp Neurol 1989;104:162–71.
84. Granholm AC, Gerhardt GA, Bygdeman M, et al. Human fetal xenografts of brainstem tissue containing locus coeruleus neurons: functional and structural studies of intraocular grafts in athymic nude rats. Exp Neurol 1992;118:7–17.
85. Tucker DC, Gist R. Sympathetic innervation alters growth and intrinsic heart rate of fetal rat atria maturing in oculo. Circ Res 1986;59:534–44.

Hypothalamic Astrocytes in Obesity

Cristina García-Cáceres, PhD[a], Chun-Xia Yi, MD, PhD[a],
Matthias H. Tschöp, MD[a,b],*

KEYWORDS

- Obesity • Hypothalamic inflammation • Astrocytes • Leptin • Insulin resistance

KEY POINTS

- Obesity is characterized by a chronic and low-grade inflammation in diverse tissues, including the hypothalamus.
- Hypothalamic inflammation is considered an early and determining factor for the onset of obesity, a factor that occurs even before body weight gain.
- Within the hypothalamus, microglia and astrocytes produce cytokines that drive inflammatory responses. Furthermore, because of their physical proximity to blood vessels and because of their function in transporting nutrients, astrocytes are directly affected by nutrient excess.
- Astrocytes might play a unique role in promoting hypothalamic inflammatory responses in obesity.

INTRODUCTION

In the last 2 decades, there has been a dramatic increase in obesity, partly because of the increased intake of energy-dense foods with a high fat content. Because excess body weight is considered an important risk factor contributing to the development of other diseases such as type 2 diabetes, hypertension, heart failure, dyslipidemia, arteriosclerosis, and cancer,[1–3] treating and reversing obesity is of paramount importance. As such, a greater understanding of the molecular mechanisms involved in the development of obesity may be the key to generating new and more effective strategies for treating this major health care problem.

Through its neural circuitry and peptides, the hypothalamus regulates food intake and energy expenditure, and impaired hypothalamic control leads to lipid accumulation and body weight gain. Numerous reports suggested that a high-fat diet (HFD) induces

[a] Institute for Diabetes and Obesity, Helmholtz Centre Munich, 85748 Garching, Munich, Germany; [b] Division of Metabolic Diseases, Department of Medicine, Technical University Munich, 81675 Munich, Germany.
* Corresponding author. Institute for Diabetes and Obesity, Business Campus Garching-Hochbrück Parkring 13, 85748 Garching, Munich, Germany.
E-mail address: matthias.tschoep@helmholtz-muenchen.de

Endocrinol Metab Clin N Am 42 (2013) 57–66
http://dx.doi.org/10.1016/j.ecl.2012.11.003
0889-8529/13/$ – see front matter © 2013 Elsevier Inc. All rights reserved.

endo.theclinics.com

chronic activation of inflammatory pathways, both in peripheral organs and within the central nervous system (CNS), including the hypothalamus.[4–14] Obese rodents exhibit increased levels of inflammatory mediators such as cytokines within metabolically relevant tissues, such as adipose tissue,[15] liver,[16] and the hypothalamus.[5,11,12] Because hypothalamic inflammation is directly linked to the development of leptin and insulin resistance, which contribute to impaired energy balance in diet-induced obese (DIO) mice,[14,17,18] the concept of hypothalamic inflammation in obesity has recently gained some attention.[5,8,12,19] The current thinking is that hypothalamic, in addition to systemic, inflammation may represent a driving factor in the development of obesity and diabetes.

HYPOTHALAMIC INFLAMMATION

A typical inflammatory response involves the production of cytokines, including tumor necrosis factor (TNF)-α and a variety of interleukins (ILs), which function in an acute manner to protect the body from damaging external influences. Metabolic stress, as can be achieved with overnutrition, can induce an inflammatory state. To this end, Thaler and colleagues[11] recently reported that a single day of HFD is sufficient to increase the hypothalamic expression of cytokines, whereas other investigators have shown that mice exposed to 3 days of HFD have abolished the ability of hypothalamic insulin to suppress white adipose tissue lipolysis and hepatic glucose production.[20] The net result of these hypothalamic inflammatory processes is thought to include leptin and insulin resistance, which results in the defective regulation of food intake during HFD feeding[5,8,14,21,22] and impaired energy balance. Because the alterations in these anorexigenic hormones occur before substantial weight gain,[5,8,11,12] it is likely that this state drives the development of obesity rather than the reverse.

Mechanisms Leading Hypothalamic Inflammation in Obesity

Several pathways are affected by HFD-induced obesity and their impairment is thought to contribute to consecutive dysregulation of hypothalamic energy balance control. Some investigators have implicated the IκB kinase-β (IKKβ)/nuclear factor-$\kappa\beta$ (NF-$\kappa\beta$) signaling pathway,[14,23,24] which mediates cellular responses to stress and inflammation. Overnutrition leads to perturbations in the endoplasmic reticulum (ER) system,[17,25] which activates IKKβ–NF-$\kappa\beta$ signaling in the hypothalamus and results in an energy imbalance.[14] It has been suggested that the role of IKKβ–NF-$\kappa\beta$ in hypothalamic insulin and leptin resistance is partly its ability to activate the expression of the suppressor of cytokine signaling (SOCS)-3,[14] a common inhibitor of leptin and insulin signaling.[21,24,26]

Toll-like receptor (TLR)-4, primarily expressed by activated microglia in DIO mice,[8] has also been shown to activate NF-$\kappa\beta$ signaling,[27] leading to disrupted leptin and insulin signaling in the hypothalamus.[8,18] Long-chain saturated fatty acids, possibly acting through TLR-4, promote the production of inflammatory cytokines, such as TNF-α, IL-1β, and IL-6,[4,28,29] which are involved in insulin resistance. These long-chain saturated fatty acids also induce ER stress in the hypothalamus.[8] The role of TLR-4 in obesity has been confirmed by diverse pharmacologic manipulations that inhibit TLR-4[18,28,30–32] and protect mice from diet-induced obesity. In contrast, the central inhibition of ER stress by phenyl butyric acid (PBA) does not lead to the reduction of hypothalamic TLR-4 expression and, thus, does not reverse diet-induced leptin resistance in the hypothalamus.[8] Thus, ER stress could be a downstream event in the cascade that ultimately triggers proinflammatory processes in the hypothalamus.[8]

Cytokines are the transcriptional targets of NF-$\kappa\beta$ activation[33] and HFD feeding has been reported to induce hypothalamic expression of cytokines TNF-α, IL-1β, and

IL-6.[5,8,11,13,18] For example, TNF-α is involved in controlling leptin and insulin signaling in the hypothalamus.[34] The central injection of a low dose of TNF-α (10^{-12} M) reproduces the effects of saturated fatty acid–induced inflammation in the hypothalamus, impairing both the secretion and action of insulin in peripheral tissues such as liver and skeletal muscle in rats.[4] Likewise, a genetic defect in either TNF-α[35,36] or its receptor[37] protects against overeating from inducing obesity or insulin resistance in mice.

Although central administration of IL-4 exacerbates hypothalamic inflammation and causes excess weight gain during HFD feeding,[38] other cytokines have antiinflammatory effects. For example, IL-6 and IL-10 seem to mediate some of the metabolic benefits of exercise. Acting on their specific receptors, expressed in most hypothalamic neurons, IL-6 and IL-10 reduce hypothalamic inflammation and improve insulin sensitivity in obese mice.[39] Acute exercise suppresses hyperphagia and hypothalamic NF-$\kappa\beta$ activation in an IL-6–dependent manner.[39] Other investigators have pointed out that IL-6 promotes inflammatory responses and insulin resistance in the hypothalamus of obese mice.[29] As already noted, HFD feeding has been reported to increase hypothalamic IL-6 expression.[5,8,11,13,18] Thus, treatment with an IL-6–neutralizing antibody leads to the restoration of the HFD-mediated inflammatory response and improves insulin action in the brain.[29]

Despite the multiple efforts to elucidate how HFD drives hypothalamic inflammation, these findings confirm the heterogeneity of mechanisms implicated in the activation of hypothalamic inflammatory responses in obesity. Such heterogeneity might result from the pleiotropic nature of cytokines,[40] different nutritional composition of HFD used, and/or individual differences in the basal metabolic and inflammatory state of an organism. Whatever the mechanism responsible, the common feature is that the hypothalamus seems to be a primary site of inflammation caused by HFD feeding, and this process may represent an early factor perpetuating the development of obesity, insulin resistance, and diabetes.[5,8,11,12]

THE ROLE OF ASTROCYTES IN HYPOTHALAMIC INFLAMMATION

As active cells in the brain,[41,42] astrocytes comodulate all aspects of neuronal function, including synaptogenesis, synaptic plasticity, neuronal metabolism and survival, homeostasis of the extracellular ionic environment and pH, and clearance and release of extracellular glutamate.[43–46] These functions are performed through direct and bidirectional communication with neurons, which is essential for normal brain function.[41,47–49]

Astrocytes are dynamic cells that respond to changes in the CNS environment by undergoing morphologic and functional alterations that are anatomically specific and that influence neuronal activities.[50,51] In response to CNS insults, astrocytes can develop a hypertrophic or reactive phenotype termed astrogliosis,[52] which is characterized by the upregulation of specific structural proteins such as glial fibrillary acidic protein (GFAP) and vimentin.[53] In response to injury, ischemia, and other stimuli, astrocytes also produce inflammatory mediators including TNF-α, IL-1β, and IL-6.[54,55] These soluble, inflammatory factors can affect neighboring cells, including microglia, neurons, and astrocytes themselves, to control the cerebral inflammatory and immune reactions (reviewed in Refs.[56,57]). Although both astrocytes and microglia are the main CNS immune-competent cells in promoting inflammatory responses in the brain (reviewed in Refs.[56,58]), astrocytes, unlike microglia, surround the endothelial cells of the blood-brain barrier (BBB)[33,59–61] and have intimate contact with both vascular and synaptic elements and with diet-derived inflammatory and metabolic factors (reviewed in Refs.[62]).

Astrocytes and microglia respond rapidly, promoting inflammation and exhibiting gliosis,[11] likely in an attempt to prevent neuronal injury, and chronic exposure to HFD could overwhelm the protective ability of glia, in which case neuronal damage and loss are no longer avoidable.[11] For example, prolonged HFD-induced hypothalamic inflammation leads to increased gliosis[11,63] associated with increased apoptosis of neurons in the hypothalamus.[7,11,22] Although the hypothalamus is dynamic in terms of hormonal sensitivity,[17,28,39] neuronal turnover,[7] gliosis,[64] and inflammation[17,65] (which can be restored after the loss of body weight induced by caloric restriction,[7] exercise,[39,64] or unsaturated fatty acids,[17] as well as by genetic and pharmacologic approaches[12,14,28,66]), often only prolonged interventions such as a low-fat feeding[13] and exercise[64] can reverse hypothalamic inflammation in obesity. Although astrocytes play a role in controlling hypothalamic inflammation induced by HFD, there remains much to be discovered with respect to how nutrient excess affects to the cytostructure of the hypothalamus and the level of involvement of astrocytes in this process.

Several lines of evidence have indicated that hypothalamic astrocytes become activated in diet-induced obesity,[11,63] and that this phenomenon occurs before substantial weight gain.[11] In obesity, astrogliosis is accompanied by increased cytokine expression[11] and the attenuation of leptin signaling in hypothalamic neurons,[67,68] suggesting a possible role of astrocytes in the regulation of leptin signaling in obesity. In DIO mice, the inhibition of hypothalamic inflammation induced by exercise[64] or unsaturated fatty acids[17] reverses microglial activation in the hypothalamus. How saturated fatty acids affect astrocytes in the hypothalamus and the physiologic and reversible nature of astrogliosis in obesity also remain to be investigated. So far, the effects of saturated fatty acids on astrocytes have been examined only in in vitro studies. Recent data have shown that saturated, but not unsaturated, fatty acids trigger the release of TNF-α and IL-6 from cultured astrocytes.[69] Furthermore, this phenomenon, induced by palmitic acid in the published experiments, does not depend on the presence of microglia and is mediated by TLR-4 and p38 and p42/44 mitogen-activated protein kinase (MAPK) activity.[69] In contrast, saturated fatty acids do not seem to induce inflammatory signaling or insulin resistance in cultured hypothalamic neurons.[70] Astrocytes are required for modulating inflammatory activities of TNF in neurons[71] and can modulate microglial activity in response to lipopolysaccharides.[72] However, other studies suggest that microglia are required for astrocytic TLR-4 expression in response to brain inflammation.[73] Still other studies have pointed out that the lack of TLR-2/TLR-4 signaling, the main effector of obesity-induced hypothalamic inflammation, attenuates IL-6 expression in cultured astrocytes. This attenuation of IL-6 expression results in enhanced levels of serine/threonine protein kinase (Akt) and glycogen synthase kinase 3 (GSK3), the intermediates of insulin signaling, either in the basal state or following insulin stimulation.[29]

Taken together, and given that reactive gliosis is often considered an early marker of diverse neurodegenerative diseases,[52,74,75] we consider that astrocytes might orchestrate the attenuation of leptin and insulin signaling and neurodegeneration in the hypothalamus through the production of a variety of inflammatory factors induced by HFD feeding (**Fig. 1**). However, in vivo approaches must be conducted to clarify the importance of astrocytes in the development of metabolic disorders such as obesity.

PARADOXIC EFFECT OF HYPOTHALAMIC INFLAMMATION IN OBESITY

Hypothalamic inflammation might exert a paradoxic effect on energy homeostasis depending on the time course, the involved specific proinflammatory signals, and

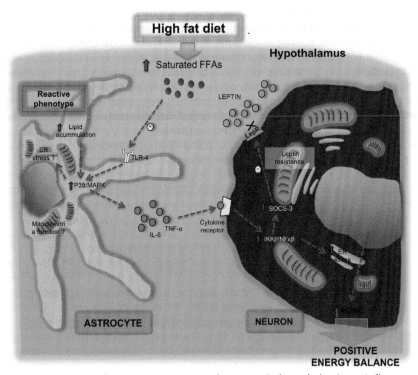

Fig. 1. Communication between astrocytes and neurons in hypothalamic proinflammatory processes leading to obesity. HFD feeding induces lipid accumulation and TLR-4 activation in astrocytes, both of which might mediate p38MAPK activity, ER stress, and the release of cytokines (IL-6 and TNF-α). These soluble inflammatory factors might be involved in the activation of IKKβ/NFκβ. IKKβ/NFκβ induces SOCS3, which suppresses leptin signaling and increases ER stress. These changes in leptin signaling reduce POMC expression, thereby promoting a positive energy balance. FFAs, free fatty acids; LepR, leptin receptor; POMC, pro-opiomelanocortin.

the degree of inflammation. Acute inflammation, at a high magnitude such as in an infection, induces a state of negative energy balance[76]; chronic, low-level inflammation, as observed in obesity, has the opposite effect.[65] The central administration of high-dose TNF-α (10^{-8} to 10^{-11} M) has catabolic effects on energy balance, increasing the metabolism of fatty acids and reducing body weight gain in mice.[4] In contrast, a low dose of TNF-α (10^{-12} M) results in a state of positive energy balance.[4,37] Studies with transgenic mice that overexpress IL-6 specifically in astrocytes (GFAP–IL-6 mice) show that these mice have chronic massive neuroinflammation, increased gliosis, oxidative stress, and neurologic disorders, but are resistant to HFD-induced increases in body weight and body fat.[77]

Hypothalamic Cytokine Signaling and Obesity

Obese rodent models are characterized by defective hypothalamic leptin signaling.[78] Leptin is a metabolic hormone but it is also structurally a cytokine and its receptor is from the same family as the IL-6 cytokine receptor.[79] Given this fact, it is possible that the chronic and low-grade inflammation induced by HFD in the hypothalamus might induce a generalized resistance not only to leptin but also to other cytokines such as IL-6, which may have physiologic significance in the hypothalamus. This resistance could be responsible for blunted activation of cytokine signaling pathways in the hypothalamus, despite the increased cytokine expression that is observed in obesity. As such, only a substantial increase in the grade of hypothalamic inflammation would reduce body weight gain and leptin resistance in DIO mice. However, such a maneuver comes at the price of cachectic outcomes, which affect not only adiposity but also lean mass of vital organs, a problem that is even more dangerous and life-threatening than obesity. This hypothesis is supported by evidence from other tissues affected by obesity-induced inflammation, such as the liver.[80] Increased hepatic inflammation following overexpression of p38 MAPK, a kinase that responds to ER stress,[80] has been reported to improve glucose metabolism in DIO and *ob/ob* mice.[81] Based on the evidence reviewed earlier, it may be useful to consider the emerging role of astrocytes in hypothalamic inflammation and cytokine signaling to develop superior therapeutic strategies for the treatment of obesity and diabetes.

REFERENCES

1. Daniels SR. Complications of obesity in children and adolescents. Int J Obes (Lond) 2009;33(Suppl 1):S60–5.
2. Tsiros MD, Olds T, Buckley JD, et al. Health-related quality of life in obese children and adolescents. Int J Obes (Lond) 2009;33(4):387–400.
3. Haslam DW, James WP. Obesity. Lancet 2005;366(9492):1197–209.
4. Arruda AP, Milanski M, Coope A, et al. Low-grade hypothalamic inflammation leads to defective thermogenesis, insulin resistance, and impaired insulin secretion. Endocrinology 2011;152(4):1314–26.
5. De Souza CT, Araujo EP, Bordin S, et al. Consumption of a fat-rich diet activates a proinflammatory response and induces insulin resistance in the hypothalamus. Endocrinology 2005;146(10):4192–9.
6. Hotamisligil GS, Arner P, Caro JF, et al. Increased adipose tissue expression of tumor necrosis factor-alpha in human obesity and insulin resistance. J Clin Invest 1995;95(5):2409–15.
7. McNay DE, Briancon N, Kokoeva MV, et al. Remodeling of the arcuate nucleus energy-balance circuit is inhibited in obese mice. J Clin Invest 2012;122(1): 142–52.
8. Milanski M, Degasperi G, Coope A, et al. Saturated fatty acids produce an inflammatory response predominantly through the activation of TLR4 signaling in hypothalamus: implications for the pathogenesis of obesity. J Neurosci 2009;29(2): 359–70.
9. Posey KA, Clegg DJ, Printz RL, et al. Hypothalamic proinflammatory lipid accumulation, inflammation, and insulin resistance in rats fed a high-fat diet. Am J Physiol Endocrinol Metab 2009;296(5):E1003–12.
10. Skinner AC, Steiner MJ, Henderson FW, et al. Multiple markers of inflammation and weight status: cross-sectional analyses throughout childhood. Pediatrics 2010;125(4):e801–9.
11. Thaler JP, Yi CX, Schur EA, et al. Obesity is associated with hypothalamic injury in rodents and humans. J Clin Invest 2012;122(1):153–62.
12. Velloso LA, Araujo EP, de Souza CT. Diet-induced inflammation of the hypothalamus in obesity. Neuroimmunomodulation 2008;15(3):189–93.
13. Wang X, Ge A, Cheng M, et al. Increased hypothalamic inflammation associated with the susceptibility to obesity in rats exposed to high-fat diet. Exp Diabetes Res 2012;2012:847246.

14. Zhang X, Zhang G, Zhang H, et al. Hypothalamic IKKbeta/NF-kappaB and ER stress link overnutrition to energy imbalance and obesity. Cell 2008;135(1):61–73.
15. Hotamisligil GS, Shargill NS, Spiegelman BM. Adipose expression of tumor necrosis factor-alpha: direct role in obesity-linked insulin resistance. Science 1993;259(5091):87–91.
16. Park EJ, Lee JH, Yu GY, et al. Dietary and genetic obesity promote liver inflammation and tumorigenesis by enhancing IL-6 and TNF expression. Cell 2010;140(2): 197–208.
17. Cintra DE, Ropelle ER, Moraes JC, et al. Unsaturated fatty acids revert diet-induced hypothalamic inflammation in obesity. PLoS One 2012;7(1):e30571.
18. Kleinridders A, Schenten D, Konner AC, et al. MyD88 signaling in the CNS is required for development of fatty acid-induced leptin resistance and diet-induced obesity. Cell Metab 2009;10(4):249–59.
19. Yi CX, Gericke M, Krüger M, et al. High calorie diet triggers hypothalamic angiopathy. Molecular Metabolism 2012. http://dx.doi.org/10.1016/j.molmet.2012.08.004.
20. Scherer T, Lindtner C, Zielinski E, et al. Short-term voluntary overfeeding disrupts brain insulin control of adipose tissue lipolysis. J Biol Chem 2012;287(39): 33061–9.
21. Howard JK, Cave BJ, Oksanen LJ, et al. Enhanced leptin sensitivity and attenuation of diet-induced obesity in mice with haploinsufficiency of Socs3. Nat Med 2004;10(7):734–8.
22. Moraes JC, Coope A, Morari J, et al. High-fat diet induces apoptosis of hypothalamic neurons. PLoS One 2009;4(4):e5045.
23. Kievit P, Howard JK, Badman MK, et al. Enhanced leptin sensitivity and improved glucose homeostasis in mice lacking suppressor of cytokine signaling-3 in POMC-expressing cells. Cell Metab 2006;4(2):123–32.
24. Mori H, Hanada R, Hanada T, et al. Socs3 deficiency in the brain elevates leptin sensitivity and confers resistance to diet-induced obesity. Nat Med 2004;10(7): 739–43.
25. Ozcan L, Ergin AS, Lu A, et al. Endoplasmic reticulum stress plays a central role in development of leptin resistance. Cell Metab 2009;9(1):35–51.
26. Ueki K, Kondo T, Kahn CR. Suppressor of cytokine signaling 1 (SOCS-1) and SOCS-3 cause insulin resistance through inhibition of tyrosine phosphorylation of insulin receptor substrate proteins by discrete mechanisms. Mol Cell Biol 2004;24(12):5434–46.
27. Hayden MS, Ghosh S. Shared principles in NF-kappaB signaling. Cell 2008; 132(3):344–62.
28. Milanski M, Arruda AP, Coope A, et al. Inhibition of hypothalamic inflammation reverses diet-induced insulin resistance in the liver. Diabetes 2012;61(6):1455–62.
29. Sartorius T, Lutz SZ, Hoene M, et al. Toll-like receptors 2 and 4 impair insulin-mediated brain activity by interleukin-6 and osteopontin and alter sleep architecture. FASEB J 2012;26(5):1799–809.
30. Poggi M, Bastelica D, Gual P, et al. C3H/HeJ mice carrying a toll-like receptor 4 mutation are protected against the development of insulin resistance in white adipose tissue in response to a high-fat diet. Diabetologia 2007;50(6):1267–76.
31. Shi H, Kokoeva MV, Inouye K, et al. TLR4 links innate immunity and fatty acid-induced insulin resistance. J Clin Invest 2006;116(11):3015–25.
32. Tsukumo DM, Carvalho-Filho MA, Carvalheira JB, et al. Loss-of-function mutation in Toll-like receptor 4 prevents diet-induced obesity and insulin resistance. Diabetes 2007;56(8):1986–98.

33. Abbott NJ. Astrocyte-endothelial interactions and blood-brain barrier permeability. J Anat 2002;200(6):629–38.

34. Moraes JC, Amaral ME, Picardi PK, et al. Inducible-NOS but not neuronal-NOS participate in the acute effect of TNF-alpha on hypothalamic insulin-dependent inhibition of food intake. FEBS Lett 2006;580(19):4625–31.

35. Ventre J, Doebber T, Wu M, et al. Targeted disruption of the tumor necrosis factor-alpha gene: metabolic consequences in obese and nonobese mice. Diabetes 1997;46(9):1526–31.

36. Uysal KT, Wiesbrock SM, Marino MW, et al. Protection from obesity-induced insulin resistance in mice lacking TNF-alpha function. Nature 1997;389(6651):610–4.

37. Romanatto T, Roman EA, Arruda AP, et al. Deletion of tumor necrosis factor-alpha receptor 1 (TNFR1) protects against diet-induced obesity by means of increased thermogenesis. J Biol Chem 2009;284(52):36213–22.

38. Oh-I S, Thaler JP, Ogimoto K, et al. Central administration of interleukin-4 exacerbates hypothalamic inflammation and weight gain during high-fat feeding. Am J Physiol Endocrinol Metab 2010;299(1):E47–53.

39. Ropelle ER, Flores MB, Cintra DE, et al. IL-6 and IL-10 anti-inflammatory activity links exercise to hypothalamic insulin and leptin sensitivity through IKKbeta and ER stress inhibition. PLoS Biol 2010;8(8). pii: e1000465.

40. Hirano T. Molecular basis underlying functional pleiotropy of cytokines and growth factors. Biochem Biophys Res Commun 1999;260(2):303–8.

41. Rakic P. Neuronal-glial interaction during brain development. Trends Neurosci 1981;4:184–7.

42. Barres BA. New roles for glia. J Neurosci 1991;11(12):3685–94.

43. Kettenmann HR, Ransom BR. Neuroglia. 2nd edition. New York: Oxford University Press; 2005.

44. Mazzanti M, Sul JY, Haydon PG. Glutamate on demand: astrocytes as a ready source. Neuroscientist 2001;7(5):396–405.

45. Pellerin L, Magistretti PJ. Neuroenergetics: calling upon astrocytes to satisfy hungry neurons. Neuroscientist 2004;10(1):53–62.

46. Ullian EM, Sapperstein SK, Christopherson KS, et al. Control of synapse number by glia. Science 2001;291(5504):657–61.

47. Pasti L, Volterra A, Pozzan T, et al. Intracellular calcium oscillations in astrocytes: a highly plastic, bidirectional form of communication between neurons and astrocytes in situ. J Neurosci 1997;17(20):7817–30.

48. Araque A, Parpura V, Sanzgiri RP, et al. Glutamate-dependent astrocyte modulation of synaptic transmission between cultured hippocampal neurons. Eur J Neurosci 1998;10(6):2129–42.

49. Araque A, Sanzgiri RP, Parpura V, et al. Astrocyte-induced modulation of synaptic transmission. Can J Physiol Pharmacol 1999;77(9):699–706.

50. Bachoo RM, Kim RS, Ligon KL, et al. Molecular diversity of astrocytes with implications for neurological disorders. Proc Natl Acad Sci U S A 2004;101(22):8384–9.

51. Hewett JA. Determinants of regional and local diversity within the astroglial lineage of the normal central nervous system. J Neurochem 2009;110(6):1717–36.

52. Levine JB, Kong J, Nadler M, et al. Astrocytes interact intimately with degenerating motor neurons in mouse amyotrophic lateral sclerosis (ALS). Glia 1999;28(3):215–24.

53. Ridet JL, Alonso G, Chauvet N, et al. Immunocytochemical characterization of a new marker of fibrous and reactive astrocytes. Cell Tissue Res 1996;283(1):39–49.

54. Lieberman AP, Pitha PM, Shin HS, et al. Production of tumor necrosis factor and other cytokines by astrocytes stimulated with lipopolysaccharide or a neurotropic virus. Proc Natl Acad Sci U S A 1989;86(16):6348–52.
55. Lee SC, Liu W, Dickson DW, et al. Cytokine production by human fetal microglia and astrocytes. Differential induction by lipopolysaccharide and IL-1 beta. J Immunol 1993;150(7):2659–67.
56. Dong Y, Benveniste EN. Immune function of astrocytes. Glia 2001;36(2):180–90.
57. Farina C, Aloisi F, Meinl E. Astrocytes are active players in cerebral innate immunity. Trends Immunol 2007;28(3):138–45.
58. Aloisi F. Immune function of microglia. Glia 2001;36(2):165–79.
59. Bradbury MW. The blood-brain barrier. Transport across the cerebral endothelium. Circ Res 1985;57(2):213–22.
60. Janzer RC, Raff MC. Astrocytes induce blood-brain barrier properties in endothelial cells. Nature 1987;325(6101):253–7.
61. Takano T, Tian GF, Peng W, et al. Astrocyte-mediated control of cerebral blood flow. Nat Neurosci 2006;9(2):260–7.
62. García-Cáceres C, Fuente-Martín E, Argente J, et al. Emerging role of glial cells in the control of body weight. Molecular Metabolism 2012. http://dx.doi.org/10.1016/j.molmet.2012.07.001.
63. Horvath TL, Sarman B, García-Cáceres C, et al. Synaptic input organization of the melanocortin system predicts diet-induced hypothalamic reactive gliosis and obesity. Proc Natl Acad Sci U S A 2010;107(33):14875–80.
64. Yi CX, Al-Massadi O, Donelan E, et al. Exercise protects against high-fat diet-induced hypothalamic inflammation. Physiol Behav 2012;106(4):485–90.
65. Thaler JP, Choi SJ, Schwartz MW, et al. Hypothalamic inflammation and energy homeostasis: resolving the paradox. Front Neuroendocrinol 2010;31(1):79–84.
66. Wisse BE, Schwartz MW. Does hypothalamic inflammation cause obesity? Cell Metab 2009;10(4):241–2.
67. Pan W, Hsuchou H, He Y, et al. Astrocyte leptin receptor (ObR) and leptin transport in adult-onset obese mice. Endocrinology 2008;149(6):2798–806.
68. Pan W, Hsuchou H, Xu C, et al. Astrocytes modulate distribution and neuronal signaling of leptin in the hypothalamus of obese A vy mice. J Mol Neurosci 2011;43(3):478–84.
69. Gupta S, Knight AG, Gupta S, et al. Saturated long-chain fatty acids activate inflammatory signaling in astrocytes. J Neurochem 2012;120(6):1060–71.
70. Choi SJ, Kim F, Schwartz MW, et al. Cultured hypothalamic neurons are resistant to inflammation and insulin resistance induced by saturated fatty acids. Am J Physiol Endocrinol Metab 2010;298(6):E1122–30.
71. Akassoglou K, Probert L, Kontogeorgos G, et al. Astrocyte-specific but not neuron-specific transmembrane TNF triggers inflammation and degeneration in the central nervous system of transgenic mice. J Immunol 1997;158(1):438–45.
72. Yang L, Tanaka J, Zhang B, et al. Astrocytes modulate nitric oxide production by microglial cells through secretion of serine and glycine. Biochem Biophys Res Commun 1998;251(1):277–82.
73. Holm TH, Draeby D, Owens T. Microglia are required for astroglial Toll-like receptor 4 response and for optimal TLR2 and TLR3 response. Glia 2012;60(4):630–8.
74. Frohman EM, van den Noort S, Gupta S. Astrocytes and intracerebral immune responses. J Clin Immunol 1989;9(1):1–9.
75. Hertz L, McFarlin DE, Waksman BH. Astrocytes: auxiliary cells for immune responses in the central nervous system? Immunol Today 1990;11(8):265–8.

76. Gautron L, Laye S. Neurobiology of inflammation-associated anorexia. Front Neurosci 2009;3:59.
77. Hidalgo J, Florit S, Giralt M, et al. Transgenic mice with astrocyte-targeted production of interleukin-6 are resistant to high-fat diet-induced increases in body weight and body fat. Brain Behav Immun 2010;24(1):119–26.
78. Munzberg H, Flier JS, Bjorbaek C. Region-specific leptin resistance within the hypothalamus of diet-induced obese mice. Endocrinology 2004;145(11):4880–9.
79. Baumann H, Morella KK, White DW, et al. The full-length leptin receptor has signaling capabilities of interleukin 6-type cytokine receptors. Proc Natl Acad Sci U S A 1996;93(16):8374–8.
80. Zarubin T, Han J. Activation and signaling of the p38 MAP kinase pathway. Cell Res 2005;15(1):11–8.
81. Lee J, Sun C, Zhou Y, et al. p38 MAPK-mediated regulation of Xbp1s is crucial for glucose homeostasis. Nat Med 2011;17(10):1251–60.

Regulation of Peripheral Metabolism by Substrate Partitioning in the Brain

Cesar Moreno, BA, BS[a], Linda Yang, PhD[b], Penny Dacks, PhD[c],
Fumiko Isoda, PhD[a], Michael Poplawski, MD, PhD[a],
Charles V. Mobbs, PhD[a],*

KEYWORDS

- Peripheral metabolism • Substrate partitioning • β-oxidation • Free fatty acids

KEY POINTS

- All organisms must adapt to changing nutrient availability, with nutrient surplus promoting glucose metabolism and nutrient deficit promoting alternative fuels (in mammals, mainly free fatty acids).
- In mammals these complex metabolic adaptations are orchestrated by nutrient-sensing neurons in the ventromedial hypothalamus.
- At least some hypothalamic neurons can metabolize free fatty acids via β-oxidation, and that β-oxidation generally opposes effects of glucose on hypothalamic neurons.
- Hypothalamic β-oxidation promotes obese phenotypes, including enhanced hepatic glucose output.
- The molecular mechanisms mediating the competition between glucose and lipid oxidation in the hypothalamus remain to be established, but probably entail regulation of the Ppar family of transcription factors.

METABOLIC FLEXIBILITY IS REQUIRED TO ADAPT TO CHANGES IN FUEL AVAILABILITY

All organisms and cell types adapt to fuel availability, although some cell types are more adaptable than others. Because glucose is the ultimate product of photosynthesis and is thus the basis of virtually all bioenergetic economy, most cell types

Funding Resources: NIH/Klarman Family Research Foundation.
Conflict of Interest: None.
[a] Department of Neuroscience, Mount Sinai School of Medicine, 1 Gustave Levy Place, New York, NY 10029, USA; [b] Beth Israel Deaconess Medical Center, Harvard Medical School, 185 Pilgrim Road, Deaconess 319, Boston, MA 02215, USA; [c] Aging & Alzheimer's Disease Prevention, Alzheimer's Drug Discovery Foundation, New York, NY 10019, USA
* Corresponding author. Department of Neuroscience, Mount Sinai School of Medicine, 1 Gustave Levy Place, New York, NY 10029.
E-mail address: charles.mobbs@mssm.edu

and organisms are optimized to use glucose to produce energy, and thus will use glucose preferentially when it is present. For example, when both glucose and lactose are present, glucose inhibits lactose metabolism, but when lactose is the sole source of carbon, lactose metabolism is induced. Indeed, studies of the molecular mechanisms by which *Escherichia coli* adapts to metabolize lactose continue to elucidate surprisingly informative mechanisms.[1–3] Yeast too will preferentially metabolize glucose, and when excess glucose is present will convert some of the glucose to ethanol in a process called fermentation, to be metabolized subsequently when glucose is no longer freely available. In animals a similar process occurs whereby glucose is the main source of energy; during the active period (in humans during the day, in rodents at night) some of the excess glucose is converted to lipid stores, then lipid stores are used by some tissues during the sleep phase or during prolonged nutritional deprivation. As with the lac operon, studies examining the mechanisms mediating these metabolic switches continue to yield surprising results.

In contrast to other cell types, neurons are relatively dependent on glucose as a source of cellular metabolism.[4] Thus the main deleterious effects of hypoglycemia encountered in diabetic patients as a result of insulin therapy are neurologic symptoms, including seizure and coma.[5,6] Because of this unique dependence, mechanisms have evolved for the brain to sense levels of blood glucose and to produce robust systemic responses to correct the level of blood glucose.

NEURONS SENSITIVE TO GLUCOSE REGULATE PERIPHERAL GLUCOSE AND LIPID HOMEOSTASIS

The earliest evidence that the brain controls levels of blood glucose was Claude Bernard's famous observation that damage to the floor of the fourth ventricle in the brain produced a rapid and sustained increase in urinary glucose.[7] Many studies have corroborated this observation with a variety of manipulations; for example, sustained elevations of blood glucose appear after many pharmacologic manipulations directed toward the brainstem.[8] Similarly, the rapid induction of hyperglycemia and feeding produced by infusing the glucose metabolism inhibitor 5-thioglucose into either the lateral or the fourth ventricle seems to be mediated, at least in part, by glucose-sensing neurons in the brainstem.[9]

On the other hand, neurons located in the ventromedial hypothalamus (VMH) have long been implicated in the control of not only blood glucose but also energy balance. Some of the earliest evidence for the function of these neurons arose from hypothalamic tumors in patients, which were observed to produce a wide variety of impairments including obesity and diabetes. Subsequent studies demonstrated that lesions in the VMH in a wide range of species produce hyperphagia, weight gain, and impaired regulation of blood glucose.[10–14] The discovery of neurons in this brain area that are uniquely sensitive to glucose[15–19] suggested that a major function of these neurons is to sense and regulate plasma glucose levels, to ensure adequate glucose supply to the brain.

As already indicated, neurons normally prefer to use glucose as their main source of energy.[4] Thus during nutritional deprivation other tissues can relatively easily adapt to use free fatty acids to produce adenosine triphosphate (ATP) via β-oxidation, while preserving glucose for utilization by neurons. A question of considerable interest is how complex organisms monitor and respond to nutritional deprivation, because impairments in this system could plausibly cause abnormalities such as obesity and diabetes when nutritional resources are not limiting. A major and conserved signal of glucose sufficiency is the insulin/insulin-like pathway, which serves this function across a wide range of species including *Caenorhabditis elegans*,[20] *Drosophila*[21] and, of course, mammals. In mammals insulin is produced by glucose-sensing pancreatic β cells and, when released, promotes glucose metabolism and lipid synthesis in relevant insulin-sensitive tissues; insulin also inhibits glucose and lipid release from relevant storage organs (mainly liver and adipocytes, respectively). Thus when glucose is readily available (usually during the active period), pancreatic β cells release insulin to promote glucose utilization and nutrient storage in the form of glycogen and lipids, and when glucose is less available (usually during the period of sleep) insulin levels drop, leading to release of glucose and lipids from storage. These direct actions of insulin were until recently thought to be the primary mediators of the switch from glucose metabolism to alternative substrates, especially free fatty acids. However, it is now appreciated that actions of insulin on hypothalamic neurons play a major role in peripheral metabolic switching.[22]

Nutritional deprivation also produces a characteristic set of neuroendocrine counterregulatory responses to preserve nutritional resources, including reduction of reproductive hormones,[23] reduced thyroid hormone,[24] reduced insulin-like growth factor (IGF)-1,[25] and increased glucocorticoids, as well as glucagon and epinephrine.[26–29] A key signal mediating these neuroendocrine responses to nutritional deprivation is the adipose-derived hormone leptin, reflecting adipose stores, acting on hypothalamic neurons expressing the leptin receptor.[30] However, it should be noted that these same neuroendocrine responses are produced when blood glucose levels decrease to less than about 2.5 mM glucose (normal blood glucose level is about 4–5 mM) even when plasma leptin and insulin are normal or even elevated.[31] Similarly, although insulin serves as a key signal to stimulate peripheral glucose disposal, insulin-induced hypoglycemia reduces peripheral glucose disposal even though insulin (and leptin) are elevated.[32]

Furthermore, fasting can induce hypothalamic responses that are independent of changes in leptin or insulin,[33] mediated at least in part by reduced glucose metabolism.[34] Indeed, hypoglycemia or 2-deoxglucose (2-DG), which blocks local glucose metabolism, mimics the neuroendocrine and metabolic responses to fasting or leptin deficiency, and these responses are independent of changes in leptin or insulin.[23,24,26]

The counterregulatory responses to hypoglycemia increase the availability of blood glucose, in part by increasing hepatic glucose production but also by reducing metabolism in peripheral organs to preserve blood glucose for brain use. VMH neurons plausibly mediate these effects on glucose metabolism because electrical stimulation of the VMH, but not the lateral hypothalamus, increases glucose metabolism in peripheral tissues, mediated by enhanced sympathetic activity.[35,36] Consistent with the results of genetic inhibition of VMH glutamate release,[37] infusion of glutamate into the VMH also enhances peripheral glucose metabolism.[36] Increased peripheral glucose metabolism from VMH stimulation does not entail increased glucose transporters, in contrast to insulin-induced glucose uptake.[38] Associated with increased glucose metabolism, VMH stimulation also increases the temperature of brown adipose tissue,[39] likely reflecting hypothalamic mediation of hypothermia induced by 2-DG.[40] Infusion of leptin specifically into the VMH also induces peripheral glucose metabolism[41] through enhancement of sympathetic nervous activity.[42]

These studies were complemented by the authors' studies demonstrating that in leptin-deficient mice, which are characterized by reduced expression of hypothalamic proopiomelanocortin (POMC),[43] transgenic restoration of POMC completely normalized blood glucose, associated with normalization of hepatic gluconeogenesis.[44]

Furthermore, infusion of glucose into the hypothalamus acutely reduces hepatic glucose output[45] as well as circulating triglycerides by reducing hepatic secretion of very low-density lipoprotein triglycerides.[46] Some effects of hypothalamic glucose in reducing hepatic glucose output may require conversion to lactate,[47] implicating a glial mechanism.[48] Taken together, these studies demonstrate that activity of glucose-sensitive hypothalamic neurons promotes peripheral glucose metabolism and reduces peripheral glucose production, especially by the liver.

This hypothesis has been substantially supported by studies from the laboratory of Sherwin and colleagues. The VMH was historically implicated as the main site of glucose-sensing neurons,[15–19] and lesions of the VMH produce diabetic[49] and obese phenotypes.[12] In this historical context the VMH, sometimes referred to as the mediobasal hypothalamus (MBH), encompassed an area including both the ventromedial nucleus (VMN) and arcuate nucleus, as well as the neuron-poor area between them, because most lesion and infusion studies could not adequately distinguish between these populations. Sherwin's group[50] also demonstrated that VMH lesions prevent the counterregulatory responses to hypoglycemia. Furthermore, localized reduction of glucose metabolism in the VMH by the metabolic inhibitor 2-DG produced a robust counterregulatory response that largely mimicked the response to whole-body hypoglycemia.[51] This study was particularly informative because the 2-DG was radiolabeled, allowing the investigators to assess the extent of spread from the infusion site. This analysis indicated that confining the 2-DG to the VMN was sufficient to produce counterregulatory responses similar to those produced by whole-body hypoglycemia.[51] Conversely, local infusion of glucose[52] or lactate[53] into the VMH blocked counterregulatory responses to whole-body hypoglycemia. These studies clearly demonstrated the key role of glucose-sensing neurons in the VMH in sensing and regulating the levels of blood glucose.

The mechanisms by which VMH neurons sense glucose leading to counterregulatory responses appear to be similar to those by which pancreatic β cells sense glucose, entailing glucose metabolism mediated by the rare pancreatic form of glucokinase.[17,19,54,55] Similarly, blocking potassium-ATP (K-ATP) channels mimics the effect of glucose in glucose-excited neurons,[17] and selectively blocking K-ATP channels in the VMH blocks counterregulatory responses to hypoglycemia, whereas activating K-ATP channels in the VMH enhances those responses. The activation of counterregulatory responses by VMH neurons seems to be mediated in part by disinhibition, because hypoglycemia reduces VMH γ-aminobutyric acid (GABA), GABA agonists block counterregulatory responses, and GABA antagonists enhance counterregulatory responses.[56] These data support the hypothesis that counterregulatory responses during hypoglycemia are mediated in part by reduced activity of glucose-stimulated GABAergic neurons in the VMH. Counterregulatory responses to hypoglycemia were also impaired by genetic inhibition of glutamate transmission, specifically the Sf-1 neurons (expressed in VMN but not arcuate nucleus).[37] Of particular importance, this study also demonstrated that blood glucose levels were also relatively lower during fasting in mice with impaired glutamate transmission, in Sf-1 neurons associated with impaired induction of hepatic gluconeogenic gene expression.[37] Because acute hypoglycemia is probably rarely encountered under normal circumstances in the wild, these observations suggest that neuroendocrine and autonomic responses to acute hypoglycemia probably reflect systems evolved to adapt to more commonly encountered caloric deficits, supporting the notion that mechanisms mediating responses to hypoglycemia and nutritional deprivation overlap (see later discussion for molecular evidence supporting this hypothesis).

FREE FATTY ACIDS ARE ROBUSTLY METABOLIZED BY THE BRAIN

As already indicated, the normal rhythms of substrate availability require metabolic adaptations of most cells to maximum glucose metabolism and lipid synthesis when glucose is available during the active period, and switch from glucose metabolism to alternative fuels, mainly free fatty acids, when nutrients are less available during the inactive/sleep period or after prolonged fasting owing to lack of nutritional resources. Historically it has been assumed that the brain is a major exception,[57] and does not metabolize free fatty acids to any significant extent and thus relies largely on glucose or ketone metabolism[58] during a prolonged fast. Several early studies infusing radiolabeled palmitate in animals fed ad libitum reported that relatively small amounts of palmitate are oxidized in vivo.[59]

More recent studies, however, have made it absolutely clear that the brain is capable of robust β-oxidation under at least some circumstances. One of the first studies to assess β-oxidation in the brain was by Geyer and colleagues,[60] who demonstrated that labeled octanoic acid was metabolized to carbon dioxide in vitro by brain slices about as efficiently as liver slices. Based on these and several other studies, a thorough review in 1961 concluded that at least in vitro brain tissue can support β-oxidation, although the importance of β-oxidation in vivo was less clear.[61] Addressing this issue, Little and colleagues[62] demonstrated that infusing radiolabeled palmitate into the brain did lead to the production of radiolabeled carbon dioxide. In fact octanoic acid is so robustly metabolized in brain that it was suggested as a marker for brain activity.[63] A widely cited article indicated that astrocytes, but not oligodendrocytes or neurons, support β-oxidation.[4] This study demonstrated that all 3 cell types metabolized ketones (acetoacetate or 3-hydroxybutyrate) at rates 7 to 9 times higher than glucose, and that astrocytes metabolized free fatty acids (octanoate and palmitate) at even higher levels than ketones.[4] As this was an in vitro study on cells derived from the developing rat, it could be argued that metabolism of these cell types is optimized for the high-fat low-carbohydrate composition of mother's milk during nursing. Nevertheless, similar metabolic demands are made on cell types during fasting in adults, and molecular evidence clearly indicates a metabolic shift in the brain away from glucose utilization and toward β-oxidation, especially in the hypothamus.[34] Similarly, ciliary neurotrophic factor robustly induces β-oxidation in astrocytes.[64] Therefore, these metabolic capabilities may not be limited to the developing stage but may be inducible by nutritional restriction.

Although it could be argued that in vitro studies may not reflect the limitations that might be encountered by free fatty acids as they cross the blood-brain barrier, there appear to be ample fatty acid transporters in the brain to allow rapid crossing of the blood-brain barrier (for example, in the choroid plexus, a major site of import for many hormones and nutrients into the brain[65]). Furthermore, radiolabeled free fatty acids rapidly equilibrate with the brain pool of fatty acid coenzyme A (CoA),[66] demonstrating that transport and metabolism of free fatty acids into the brain occurs rapidly and robustly. Similarly, radiolabeled octanoate, myristic acid, and linoleic acid rapidly cross the blood-brain barrier in adults.[67] Another study indicated that about 50% of palmitic acid that enters the brain is metabolized by β-oxidation.[68] More definitely, Ebert and colleagues[69] demonstrated with nuclear magnetic resonance that the metabolism of octanoate, one of the most abundant free fatty acids in the blood, constitutes as much as 20% of total brain oxidative metabolism. One reason that early studies may not have detected significant brain β-oxidation from some substrates may be that the studies were carried out in animals fed ad libitum, whereas fasting significantly increases the transport of free fatty acids across the blood-brain barrier.[70]

FREE FATTY ACIDS OPPOSE EFFECTS OF GLUCOSE ON THE ACTIVITY OF HYPOTHALAMIC NEURONS

One of the first reports indicating that hypothalamic neurons sense lipids was by Oomura and colleagues[71] (who also discovered that hypothalamic neurons sense glucose). This study indicated that free fatty acids (palmitate and oleic acid) produce effects on neurons opposite to those of glucose on glucose-inhibited neurons in the lateral hypothalamus and glucose-excited neurons in the ventromedial hypothalamus.[71] These observations were consistent with the normal physiology of the system, because increased glucose is normally a signal of nutritional sufficiency and free fatty acids are normally elevated during nutritional deprivation (an exception is the consumption of high-fat meals, which in most species including humans is mainly a modern phenomenon with pathologic consequences, as discussed later). Thus, for instance, exemplifying a general if not universal biochemical principle of substrate competition,[3] free fatty acids and glucose inhibit the metabolism of each other.[72] Therefore, it would be expected that these 2 types of nutrients would produce opposite effects on neurons whose function is to monitor nutritional status and regulate metabolic function accordingly. Nevertheless, subsequent reports indicated a much more complex relationship between the effects of glucose and effects of free fatty acids on hypothalamic neurons.[73] Some of these differences could be attributable to different concentrations of glucose and free fatty acids used to assess the responsiveness of hypothalamic neurons. Subsequent in vivo studies suggested that oleic acid in the hypothalamus inhibits glucose production and food intake via activation of K-ATP channels.[74] Although activation of K-ATP channels would be expected to oppose effects of glucose in hypothalamic neurons, consistent with the opposing effects reported by Oomura and colleagues,[71] effects on glucose production were not consistent with the hypothesis that free fatty acids serve as a signal for nutritional deprivation. Contributing to the lack of clarity in the field was the question of whether free fatty acids were sensed by hypothalamic neurons via metabolism, as is the case for glucose, or possibly through a cell-surface receptor such as FAT/CD36.[75] One study suggested that both β-oxidation and nonmetabolic effects contribute to the electrical effects of palmitate on hypothalamic neurons.[75]

Because the brain has historically not been thought to support significant metabolism of free fatty acids by β-oxidation,[57] and because there are many kinds of free fatty acids, there had been few studies addressing the functional significance of hypothalamic β-oxidation in regulating peripheral metabolism. It is thus perhaps not surprising that one of the first studies clearly implicating hypothalamic β-oxidation in regulating peripheral metabolism arose through serendipity. Loftus and colleagues[76] had developed inhibitors of fatty acid synthase as possible treatments for cancer, based on the hypothesis that cancer cells might require relatively elevated levels of fatty acid synthesis. Although these inhibitors exhibited relatively limited antitumor activity, one, C75, produced profound anorexia.[76] Normally anorexia would be considered an undesirable and common iatrogenic effect of a novel drug, but to the credit of these investigators they assessed the mechanism mediating the anorectic effect. These studies revealed that C75 produced anorexia by enhancing the levels of hypothalamic malonyl CoA.[76] The classic effect of malonyl CoA (produced by and serving as a signal for glucose metabolism) in the periphery is to block the enzyme carnitine palmitoyl transferase (Cpt1), especially the liver isoform Cpt1a, and thus block metabolism of free fatty acids by β-oxidation.[77] Based on these observations, Ruderman and colleagues[77] hypothesized that this mechanism may also occur in hypothalamic neurons expressing glucokinase. Loftus and colleagues[76] concluded that their studies with C75 supported this hypothesis. Thus despite the general consensus that the brain does not support significant β-oxidation,[57] these studies clearly indicated that β-oxidation in the hypothalamus plays an essential role in regulating energy balance, particularly in glucose-sensing neurons, which the authors have demonstrated to express the pancreatic form of glucokinase,[17,78] later corroborated by more extensive analysis.[19]

In a series of studies, these investigators and their colleagues further corroborated the importance of hypothalamic malonyl CoA in regulating energy balance and glucose homeostasis.[79–85] For example, they demonstrated that fasting decreases hypothalamic malonyl CoA (thus increasing hypothalamic β-oxidation), whereas feeding rapidly increases hypothalamic malonyl CoA.[82] As expected, intracerebroventricular infusion of C75 caused a rapid increase in malonyl CoA, and preventing this rapid increase blocked effects of C75, including the reduction of hypothalamic agouti-related peptide (AgRP) and neuropeptide Y and an increase in hypothalamic POMC, both of which plausibly mediate effects of C75 on energy balance.[82] Of particular interest, central administration of C75 induced a rapid increase in skeletal β-oxidation, mediated by sympathetic activation of skeletal Ppar-α,[86] which promotes β-oxidation. Some effects of leptin may also depend on hypothalamic β-oxidation, because blocking the effect of leptin to increase hypothalamic acetyl-CoA carboxylase (which synthesizes malonyl CoA) blocks the effects of leptin.[87]

The importance of hypothalamic β-oxidation in regulating glucose homeostasis was subsequently confirmed by Obici and colleagues,[88] who demonstrated that inhibiting hypothalamic Cpt1a (which they called Cpt1L, for the liver form) reduced food intake and hepatic glucose output. Similarly, experimental enhancement of hypothalamic malonyl-CoA decarboxylase, which degrades malonyl CoA, thus activating hypothalamic β-oxidation, leads to obese phenotypes and impaired glucose homeostasis.[85,89] Furthermore, pro-obesity phenotypes produced by the hormone ghrelin are blocked by inhibition of hypothalamic Cpt1a.[90–92]

Interest in the role of hypothalamic β-oxidation arose from examination of hypothalamic molecular responses to hypoglycemia and fasting, which preliminary studies suggested entailed induction of hypothalamic Cpt1a (but not Cpt1c) and reduction in glycolysis.[93] While assessing molecular mechanisms mediating the suppression of counterregulation by estradiol, the authors observed that estradiol inhibited hypothalamic Cpt1a, plausibly contributing to counterregulatory failure by increasing reliance on glycolysis.[94] Similarly, it was observed that repetitive hypoglycemia also reduced hypothalamic expression of Cpt1a in association with counterregulatory failure.[95] The authors also confirmed the induction of Cpt1a by fasting in the hypothalamus, but not the cortex.[34] β-Oxidation is likely particularly important in POMC and AgRP neurons, which produce peroxisomes that support β-oxidation.[96] Finally, the authors have corroborated the results of Obici and colleagues and have demonstrated that chronically enhanced expression of hypothalamic Cpt1a via adeno-associated virus (AAV)-mediated gene transfer produces robust obese phenotypes, including hyperphagia and enhanced blood glucose (Yang and colleagues, 2012).

Thus although historically the brain was thought not to support β-oxidation, there is now overwhelming support that even human brains support β-oxidation under certain conditions, including type 1 diabetes and nutritional deprivation.[97] In vivo studies consistently demonstrate that hypothalamic β-oxidation is associated with obese phenotypes, such that conditions that either directly[88] or indirectly[76,79–85,89,98] reduce β-oxidation reduce obese phenotypes, whereas increasing hypothalamic β-oxidation promotes obese phenotypes (Yang and colleagues, 2012). Thus in vivo studies suggest that hypothalamic lipid metabolism serves as a signal for nutritional deprivation, consistent with early reports that lipids and glucose produce opposite effects on hypothalamic glucose-sensing neurons,[71] agreeing with molecular evidence that fasting induces β-oxidation.[34] Later in vitro studies were not as consistent, probably because effects of free fatty acids on hypothalamic neuronal activity are highly dependent on ambient glucose concentrations.[99]

Although astrocytes robustly support β-oxidation, there is less evidence that neurons support β-oxidation.[4] Nevertheless, peroxisomes are expressed in specific neuronal populations in the hypothalamus, including POMC and AgRP neurons, with more peroxisomes associated with obese phenotypes.[96] Furthermore, enhanced hypothalamic expression of malonyl-CoA decarboxylase produced obese phenotypes, apparently by enhancing hypothalamic β-oxidation.[89] Because this gene was transferred using a neurotropic AAV vector, it is highly likely that its effects were mediated by neurons, and thus on neuronal β-oxidation. Using a similar AAV vector, the authors have also observed that direct activation of β-oxidation by enhanced expression of Cpt1a targeted to the VMN produces obese phenotypes, again almost certainly via actions on neuronal β-oxidation (Yang and colleagues, 2012). It is plausible, as has been previously proposed,[77] that β-oxidation in neurons may be largely confined to neurons that function to sense nutrient state and regulate peripheral metabolism, for example, glucokinase-expressing glucose-sensing neurons,[17,19] which also largely overlap with neurons sensitive to leptin.[34]

The molecular mechanisms mediating the effects of free fatty acids on hypothalamic function remain to be determined. As already suggested, hypoglycemia produces metabolic[31] and molecular[95] effects similar to those produced by fasting.[34,100] In turn, metabolic responses to fasting require Ppar-α.[100–103] Therefore, mice in which Ppar-α has been ablated exhibit relative hypoglycemia after an overnight fast.[101] The control of glucose metabolism by Ppar-α is mediated by the brain, not the liver.[104,105] For example, replacing Ppar-α in the liver of Ppar-α knockout mice does not reverse the elevated whole-body glucose metabolism in these mice, but activating Ppar-α in the brain reduces whole-body glucose metabolism.[104] This observation led the investigators to conclude that "the alteration in adipocyte glucose metabolism in the knockout mice may result from the absence of Ppar-α in the brain."[104] Similarly, pharmacologic activation of Ppar-α specifically in the hypothalamus reverses peripheral hypoglycemia observed in FASKO mice.[105] Likewise, many responses to fasting are mediated by hypothalamic neurons through leptin signaling,[30] which in turn depends on glucose metabolism.[34,106] The authors have recently reported that acute hypoglycemia induces many genes in the hypothalamus that are targets of the transcription factor Ppar-α, and the induction of these genes is correlated with endocrine responses.[95] These observations led to the hypothesis that many whole-body responses to hypoglycemia and fasting are mediated by Ppar-α in the VMH.[95] Because Ppar-α activity is induced by free fatty acids, and nutrient sensing in hypothalamic neurons controls peripheral Ppar-α gene expression and corresponding target genes via the sympathetic nervous system,[86] these observations suggest that hypothalamic free fatty acids may produce peripheral responses to fasting via induction of peripheral Ppar-α.

A major question is how hypothalamic β-oxidation promotes obese phenotypes and increases peripheral glucose homeostasis. In a series of studies, Rossetti's group[74,88,89,107,108] supported the hypothesis that hypothalamic β-oxidation enhances hepatic glucose output by metabolizing long-chain fatty acids, including oleic acid. Conversely, the same investigators argued that hypothalamic oleic acid reduces the output of hepatic glucose by activation of hypothalamic K-ATP channels.[74,88,89,107,108] Though attractive, this hypothesis poses some problems. For example, under ordinary circumstances, certainly in rodents in which these studies were done, circulating levels of free fatty acids are elevated during the fasted state and reduced in the fed state.[109,110] The exception to this circumstance would be consumption of a high-fat diet. However, both circumstances promote, rather than reduce, obese phenotypes and hepatic glucose output. On the other hand, some evidence supports that hypothalamic β-oxidation promotes obese phenotypes by reducing hypothalamic glucose sensing,[111] consistent with substrate competition observed in the periphery.[77] Furthermore, promotion of obese phenotypes by hypothalamic β-oxidation appears to be mediated by a reduction in reactive oxygen species,[96] consistent with a reduction in glucose metabolism.[112] Of course these two mechanisms are not necessarily mutually exclusive and could be linked if long-chain fatty acids such as oleic acid enhance glucose metabolism. On the other hand, oleic acid and glucose produce opposite effects on K-ATP channel function (consistent with the opposing actions of these nutrients in many systems), while apparently having the same effect on output of hepatic glucose. Further studies will be required to resolve these apparent inconsistencies.

REFERENCES

1. Ozbudak EM, Thattai M, Lim HN, et al. Multistability in the lactose utilization network of *Escherichia coli*. Nature 2004;427(6976):737–40.
2. Lewis M. The lac repressor. C R Biol 2005;328(6):521–48.
3. Mobbs CV, Mastaitis JW, Zhang M, et al. Secrets of the lac operon. Glucose hysteresis as a mechanism in dietary restriction, aging and disease. Interdiscip Top Gerontol 2007;35:39–68.
4. Edmond J, Robbins RA, Bergstrom JD, et al. Capacity for substrate utilization in oxidative metabolism by neurons, astrocytes, and oligodendrocytes from developing brain in primary culture. J Neurosci Res 1987;18(4):551–61.
5. Cryer PE, Fisher JN, Shamoon H. Hypoglycemia. Diabetes Care 1994;17(7): 734–55.
6. Mohseni S. Hypoglycemic neuropathy. Acta Neuropathol 2001;102(5):413–21.
7. Bernard C. Influence de la section des pédoncules cérébelleux moyens sur la composition de l'urine. CR Soc Biol 1849. p. 14.
8. Feldberg W, Pyke D, Stubbs WA. Hyperglycaemia: imitating Claude Bernard's piqure with drugs. J Auton Nerv Syst 1985;14(3):213–28.
9. Ritter RC, Slusser PG, Stone S. Glucoreceptors controlling feeding and blood glucose: location in the hindbrain. Science 1981;213(4506):451–2.
10. Hetherington AW, Ranson SW. Hypothalamic lesions and adiposity in the rat. Anat Rec 1940;78:149–72.
11. Debons AF, Krimsky I. Regulation of food intake: role of the ventromedial hypothalamus. Postgrad Med 1972;51(5):74–8.
12. Goldman JK, MacKenzie R, Bernardis LL, et al. Early metabolic changes following destruction of the ventromedial hypothalamic nuclei. Metabolism 1980;29(11):1061–4.
13. Komeda K, Yokote M, Oki Y. Diabetic syndrome in the Chinese hamster induced with monosodium glutamate. Experientia 1980;36(2):232–4.
14. Bergen HT, Monkman N, Mobbs CV. Injection with gold thioglucose impairs sensitivity to glucose: evidence that glucose-responsive neurons are important for long-term regulation of body weight. Brain Res 1996;734(1–2):332–6.
15. Oomura Y, Ono T, Ooyama H, et al. Glucose and osmosensitive neurones of the rat hypothalamus. Nature 1969;222(190):282–4.

16. Orzi F, Lucignani G, Dow-Edwards D, et al. Local cerebral glucose utilization in controlled graded levels of hyperglycemia in the conscious rat. J Cereb Blood Flow Metab 1988;8(3):346–56.

17. Yang XJ, Kow LM, Funabashi T, et al. Hypothalamic glucose sensor: similarities to and differences from pancreatic beta-cell mechanisms. Diabetes 1999;48(9): 1763–72.

18. Song Z, Levin BE, McArdle JJ, et al. Convergence of pre- and postsynaptic influences on glucosensing neurons in the ventromedial hypothalamic nucleus. Diabetes 2001;50(12):2673–81.

19. Dunn-Meynell AA, Routh VH, Kang L, et al. Glucokinase is the likely mediator of glucosensing in both glucose-excited and glucose-inhibited central neurons. Diabetes 2002;51(7):2056–65.

20. Kimura KD, Tissenbaum HA, Liu Y, et al. daf-2, an insulin receptor-like gene that regulates longevity and diapause in *Caenorhabditis elegans*. Science 1997; 277(5328):942–6.

21. Clancy DJ, Gems D, Harshman LG, et al. Extension of life-span by loss of CHICO, a *Drosophila* insulin receptor substrate protein. Science 2001;292(5514):104–6.

22. Scherer T, O'Hare J, Diggs-Andrews K, et al. Brain insulin controls adipose tissue lipolysis and lipogenesis. Cell Metab 2011;13(2):183–94.

23. Nagatani S, Bucholtz DC, Murahashi K, et al. Reduction of glucose availability suppresses pulsatile luteinizing hormone release in female and male rats. Endocrinology 1996;137(4):1166–70.

24. Schultes B, Oltmanns KM, Kern W, et al. Acute and prolonged effects of insulin-induced hypoglycemia on the pituitary-thyroid axis in humans. Metabolism 2002;51(10):1370–4.

25. Fontana L, Klein S, Holloszy JO. Effects of long-term calorie restriction and endurance exercise on glucose tolerance, insulin action, and adipokine production. Age (Dordr) 2010;32(1):97–108.

26. Heller SR, Cryer PE. Reduced neuroendocrine and symptomatic responses to subsequent hypoglycemia after 1 episode of hypoglycemia in nondiabetic humans. Diabetes 1991;40(2):223–6.

27. Maggs DG, Sherwin RS. Mechanisms of the sympathoadrenal response to hypoglycemia. Adv Pharmacol 1998;42:622–6.

28. Baker D, Evans M, Cryer P, et al. Hypoglycemia and glucose sensing. Diabetologia 1997;40:B83–8.

29. Cryer PE. Hierarchy of physiological responses to hypoglycemia: relevance to clinical hypoglycemia in type I (insulin dependent) diabetes mellitus. Horm Metab Res 1997;29(3):92–6.

30. Ahima RS, Flier JS. Leptin. Annu Rev Physiol 2000;62:413–37.

31. Hoffman RP. Sympathetic mechanisms of hypoglycemic counterregulation. Curr Diabetes Rev 2007;3(3):185–93.

32. Cohen N, Rossetti L, Shlimovich P, et al. Counterregulation of hypoglycemia. Skeletal muscle glycogen metabolism during three hours of physiological hyperinsulinemia in humans. Diabetes 1995;44(4):423–30.

33. Mizuno TM, Makimura H, Silverstein J, et al. Fasting regulates hypothalamic neuropeptide Y, agouti-related peptide, and proopiomelanocortin in diabetic mice independent of changes in leptin or insulin. Endocrinology 1999;140(10): 4551–7.

34. Poplawski MM, Mastaitis JW, Yang XJ, et al. Hypothalamic responses to fasting indicate metabolic reprogramming away from glycolysis toward lipid oxidation. Endocrinology 2010;151(11):5206–17.

35. Takahashi A, Shimazu T. Hypothalamic regulation of lipid metabolism in the rat: effect of hypothalamic stimulation on lipogenesis. J Auton Nerv Syst 1982;6(2): 225–35.

36. Sudo M, Minokoshi Y, Shimazu T. Ventromedial hypothalamic stimulation enhances peripheral glucose uptake in anesthetized rats. Am J Physiol 1991; 261(3 Pt 1):E298–303.

37. Tong Q, Ye C, McCrimmon RJ, et al. Synaptic glutamate release by ventromedial hypothalamic neurons is part of the neurocircuitry that prevents hypoglycemia. Cell Metab 2007;5(5):383–93.

38. Shimazu T, Sudo M, Minokoshi Y, et al. Role of the hypothalamus in insulin-independent glucose uptake in peripheral tissues. Brain Res Bull 1991; 27(3–4):501–4.

39. Minokoshi Y, Okano Y, Shimazu T. Regulatory mechanism of the ventromedial hypothalamus in enhancing glucose uptake in skeletal muscles. Brain Res 1994;649(1–2):343–7.

40. Pelz KM, Routman D, Driscoll JR, et al. Monosodium glutamate-induced arcuate nucleus damage affects both natural torpor and 2DG-induced torpor-like hypo-thermia in Siberian hamsters. Am J Physiol Regul Integr Comp Physiol 2008; 294(1):R255–65.

41. Minokoshi Y, Haque MS, Shimazu T. Microinjection of leptin into the ventromedial hypothalamus increases glucose uptake in peripheral tissues in rats. Diabetes 1999;48(2):287–91.

42. Haque MS, Minokoshi Y, Hamai M, et al. Role of the sympathetic nervous system and insulin in enhancing glucose uptake in peripheral tissues after intrahypotha-lamic injection of leptin in rats. Diabetes 1999;48(9):1706–12.

43. Mizuno TM, Kleopoulos SP, Bergen HT, et al. Rapid Communication: hypotha-lamic pro-opiomelanocortin mRNA is reduced by fasting and in ob/ob and db/db mice, but is stimulated by leptin. Diabetes 1998;47(2):294–7.

44. Mizuno TM, Kelly K, Pasinetti GM, et al. Transgenic neuronal expression of proo-piomelanocortin attenuates fasting-induced hyperphagia and reverses meta-bolic impairments in leptin-deficient obese mice. Diabetes 2003;52(11):2675–83.

45. Lam TK, Gutierrez-Juarez R, Pocai A, et al. Regulation of blood glucose by hypothalamic pyruvate metabolism. Science 2005;309(5736):943–7.

46. Lam TK, Gutierrez-Juarez R, Pocai A, et al. Brain glucose metabolism controls the hepatic secretion of triglyceride-rich lipoproteins. Nat Med 2007;13(2): 171–80.

47. Kokorovic A, Cheung GW, Rossetti L, et al. Hypothalamic sensing of circulating lactate regulates glucose production. J Cell Mol Med 2009;13(11–12):4403–8.

48. Tsacopoulos M, Magistretti PJ. Metabolic coupling between glia and neurons. J Neurosci 1996;16(3):877–85.

49. Shimazu T, Fukuda A, Ban T. Reciprocal influences of the ventromedial and lateral hypothalamic nuclei on blood glucose level and liver glycogen content. Nature 1966;210(41):1178–9.

50. Borg WP, During MJ, Sherwin RS, et al. Ventromedial hypothalamic lesions in rats suppress counterregulatory responses to hypoglycemia. J Clin Invest 1994;93(4):1677–82.

51. Borg WP, Sherwin RS, During MJ, et al. Local ventromedial hypothalamus gluco-penia triggers counterregulatory hormone release. Diabetes 1995;44(2):180–4.

52. Borg MA, Sherwin RS, Borg WP, et al. Local ventromedial hypothalamus glucose perfusion blocks counterregulation during systemic hypoglycemia in awake rats. J Clin Invest 1997;99(2):361–5.

53. Borg MA, Tamborlane WV, Shulman GI, et al. Local lactate perfusion of the ventromedial hypothalamus suppresses hypoglycemic counterregulation. Diabetes 2003;52(3):663–6.

54. Sanders NM, Dunn-Meynell AA, Levin BE. Third ventricular alloxan reversibly impairs glucose counterregulatory responses. Diabetes 2004;53(5):1230–6.

55. Levin BE, Becker TC, Eiki J, et al. Ventromedial hypothalamic glucokinase is an important mediator of the counterregulatory response to insulin-induced hypoglycemia. Diabetes 2008;57(5):1371–9.

56. Chan O, Lawson M, Zhu W, et al. ATP-sensitive K(+) channels regulate the release of GABA in the ventromedial hypothalamus during hypoglycemia. Diabetes 2007;56(4):1120–6.

57. Speijer D. Oxygen radicals shaping evolution: why fatty acid catabolism leads to peroxisomes while neurons do without it: FADH/NADH flux ratios determining mitochondrial radical formation were crucial for the eukaryotic invention of peroxisomes and catabolic tissue differentiation. Bioessays 2011;33(2):88–94.

58. Owen OE, Morgan AP, Kemp HG, et al. Brain metabolism during fasting. J Clin Invest 1967;46(10):1589–95.

59. Allweis C, Landau T, Abeles M, et al. The oxidation of uniformly labelled albumin-bound palmitic acid to CO_2 by the perfused cat brain. J Neurochem 1966;13(9): 795–804.

60. Geyer RP, Matthews LW, Stare FJ. Metabolism of emulsified trilaurin (-C1400-) and octanoic acid (-C1400-) by rat tissue slices. J Biol Chem 1949;180(3): 1037–45.

61. Fritz IB. Factors influencing the rates of long-chain fatty acid oxidation and synthesis in mammalian systems. Physiol Rev 1961;41:52–129.

62. Little JR, Hori S, Spitzer JJ. Oxidation of radioactive palmitate and glucose infused into the cortical subarachnoid space. Am J Physiol 1969;217(4):919–22.

63. Rowley H, Collins RC. [1-14C]Octanoate: a fast functional marker of brain activity. Brain Res 1985;335(2):326–9.

64. Escartin C, Pierre K, Colin A, et al. Activation of astrocytes by CNTF induces metabolic plasticity and increases resistance to metabolic insults. J Neurosci 2007;27(27):7094–104.

65. Ho HT, Dahlin A, Wang J. Expression profiling of solute carrier gene families at the blood-CSF barrier. Front Pharmacol 2012;3:154.

66. Rapoport SI. In vivo labeling of brain phospholipids by long-chain fatty acids: relation to turnover and function. Lipids 1996;31(Suppl):S97–101.

67. Spector R. Fatty acid transport through the blood-brain barrier. J Neurochem 1988;50(2):639–43.

68. Miller JC, Gnaedinger JM, Rapoport SI. Utilization of plasma fatty acid in rat brain: distribution of [14C]palmitate between oxidative and synthetic pathways. J Neurochem 1987;49(5):1507–14.

69. Ebert D, Haller RG, Walton ME. Energy contribution of octanoate to intact rat brain metabolism measured by 13C nuclear magnetic resonance spectroscopy. J Neurosci 2003;23(13):5928–35.

70. Ishiwata K, Ishii K, Ogawa K, et al. A brain uptake study of [1-(11)C]hexanoate in the mouse: the effect of hypoxia, starvation and substrate competition. Ann Nucl Med 1996;10(2):265–70.

71. Oomura Y, Nakamura T, Sugimori M, et al. Effect of free fatty acid on the rat lateral hypothalamic neurons. Physiol Behav 1975;14(04):483–6.

72. Randle PJ. Regulatory interactions between lipids and carbohydrates: the glucose fatty acid cycle after 35 years. Diabetes Metab Rev 1998;14(4):263–83.

73. Le Foll C, Irani BG, Magnan C, et al. Characteristics and mechanisms of hypo-thalamic neuronal fatty acid sensing. Am J Physiol Regul Integr Comp Physiol 2009;297(3):R655–64.

74. Obici S, Feng Z, Morgan K, et al. Central administration of oleic acid inhibits glucose production and food intake. Diabetes 2002;51(2):271–5.

75. Migrenne S, Le Foll C, Levin BE, et al. Brain lipid sensing and nervous control of energy balance. Diabetes Metab 2011;37(2):83–8.

76. Loftus TM, et al. Reduced food intake and body weight in mice treated with fatty acid synthase inhibitors. Science 2000;288(5475):2379–81.

77. Ruderman NB, Saha AK, Vavvas D, et al. Malonyl-CoA, fuel sensing, and insulin resistance. Am J Physiol 1999;276(1 Pt 1):E1–18.

78. Yang XJ, Kow LM, Pfaff DW, et al. Metabolic pathways that mediate inhibition of hypothalamic neurons by glucose. Diabetes 2004;53(1):67–73.

79. Pizer ES, Thupari J, Han WF, et al. Malonyl-coenzyme-A is a potential mediator of cytotoxicity induced by fatty-acid synthase inhibition in human breast cancer cells and xenografts. Cancer Res 2000;60(2):213–8.

80. Kumar MV, Shimokawa T, Nagy TR, et al. Differential effects of a centrally acting fatty acid synthase inhibitor in lean and obese mice. Proc Natl Acad Sci U S A 2002;99(4):1921–5.

81. Shimokawa T, Kumar MV, Lane MD. Effect of a fatty acid synthase inhibitor on food intake and expression of hypothalamic neuropeptides. Proc Natl Acad Sci U S A 2002;99(1):66–71.

82. Hu Z, Cha SH, Chohnan S, et al. Hypothalamic malonyl-CoA as a mediator of feeding behavior. Proc Natl Acad Sci U S A 2003;100(22):12624–9.

83. Kim EK, Miller I, Aja S, et al. C75, a fatty acid synthase inhibitor, reduces food intake via hypothalamic AMP-activated protein kinase. J Biol Chem 2004;279(19):19970–6.

84. Landree LE, Hanlon AL, Strong DW, et al. C75, a fatty acid synthase inhibitor, modulates AMP-activated protein kinase to alter neuronal energy metabolism. J Biol Chem 2004;279(5):3817–27.

85. Hu Z, Dai Y, Prentki M, et al. A role for hypothalamic malonyl-CoA in the control of food intake. J Biol Chem 2005;280(48):39681–3.

86. Cha SH, Hu Z, Chohnan S, et al. Inhibition of hypothalamic fatty acid synthase triggers rapid activation of fatty acid oxidation in skeletal muscle. Proc Natl Acad Sci U S A 2005;102(41):14557–62.

87. Gao S, Kinzig KP, Aja S, et al. Leptin activates hypothalamic acetyl-CoA carbox-ylase to inhibit food intake. Proc Natl Acad Sci U S A 2007;104(44):17358–63.

88. Obici S, Feng Z, Arduini A, et al. Inhibition of hypothalamic carnitine palmitoyltransferase-1 decreases food intake and glucose production. Nat Med 2003;9(6):756–61.

89. He W, Lam TK, Obici S, et al. Molecular disruption of hypothalamic nutrient sensing induces obesity. Nat Neurosci 2006;9(2):227–33.

90. Andrews ZB, Liu ZW, Walllingford N, et al. UCP2 mediates ghrelin's action on NPY/AgRP neurons by lowering free radicals. Nature 2008;454(7206):846–51.

91. Lopez M, Lage R, Saha AK, et al. Hypothalamic fatty acid metabolism mediates the orexigenic action of ghrelin. Cell Metab 2008;7(5):389–99.

92. Lage R, Vazquez MJ, Varela L, et al. Ghrelin effects on neuropeptides in the rat hypothalamus depend on fatty acid metabolism actions on BSX but not on gender. FASEB J 2010;24:2670–9.

93. Mobbs CV, Yen K, Mastaitis J, et al. Mining microarrays for metabolic meaning: nutritional regulation of hypothalamic gene expression. Neurochem Res 2004; 29(6):1093–103.

94. Cheng H, Isoda F, Mobbs CV. Estradiol impairs hypothalamic molecular responses to hypoglycemia. Brain Res 2009;1280:77–83.

95. Poplawski MM, Mastaitis JW, Mobbs CV. Naloxone, but not valsartan, preserves responses to hypoglycemia after antecedent hypoglycemia: role of metabolic reprogramming in counterregulatory failure. Diabetes 2011;60(1):39–46.

96. Diano S, Liu ZW, Jeong JK, et al. Peroxisome proliferation-associated control of reactive oxygen species sets melanocortin tone and feeding in diet-induced obesity. Nat Med 2011;17(9):1121–7.

97. Page KA, Williamson A, Yu N, et al. Medium-chain fatty acids improve cognitive function in intensively treated type 1 diabetic patients and support in vitro synaptic transmission during acute hypoglycemia. Diabetes 2009;58(5):1237–44.

98. Kuhajda FP, Pizer ES, Li JN, et al. Synthesis and antitumor activity of an inhibitor of fatty acid synthase. Proc Natl Acad Sci U S A 2000;97(7):3450–4.

99. Levin BE, Magnan C, Dunn-Meynell A, et al. Metabolic sensing and the brain: who, what, where, and how? Endocrinology 2011;152(7):2552–7.

100. Makowski L, Noland RC, Koves TR, et al. Metabolic profiling of PPARalpha-/-mice reveals defects in carnitine and amino acid homeostasis that are partially reversed by oral carnitine supplementation. FASEB J 2009;23(2):586–604.

101. Xu J, Xiao G, Trujillo C, et al. Peroxisome proliferator-activated receptor alpha (PPARalpha) influences substrate utilization for hepatic glucose production. J Biol Chem 2002;277(52):50237–44.

102. Xu J, Chang V, Joseph SB, et al. Peroxisomal proliferator-activated receptor alpha deficiency diminishes insulin-responsiveness of gluconeogenic/glycolytic/pentose gene expression and substrate cycle flux. Endocrinology 2004; 145(3):1087–95.

103. Vaitheesvaran B, Chueh FY, Xu J, et al. Advantages of dynamic "closed loop" stable isotope flux phenotyping over static "open loop" clamps in detecting silent genetic and dietary phenotypes. Metabolomics 2010;6(2):180–90.

104. Knauf C, Rieusset J, Foretz M, et al. Peroxisome proliferator-activated receptor-alpha-null mice have increased white adipose tissue glucose utilization, GLUT4, and fat mass: role in liver and brain. Endocrinology 2006;147(9):4067–78.

105. Chakravarthy MV, Zhu Y, Lopez M, et al. Brain fatty acid synthase activates PPARalpha to maintain energy homeostasis. J Clin Invest 2007;117(9):2539–52.

106. Su H, Jiang L, Carter-Su C, et al. Glucose enhances leptin signaling through modulation of AMPK activity. PLoS One 2012;7(2):e31636.

107. Lam TK, Schwartz GJ, Rossetti L. Hypothalamic sensing of fatty acids. Nat Neurosci 2005;8(5):579–84.

108. Pocai A, Lam TK, Obici S, et al. Restoration of hypothalamic lipid sensing normalizes energy and glucose homeostasis in overfed rats. J Clin Invest 2006;116(4):1081–91.

109. Richieri GV, Kleinfeld AM. Unbound free fatty acid levels in human serum. J Lipid Res 1995;36(2):229–40.

110. Sonnenberg GE, Krakower GR, Hoffmann RG, et al. Plasma leptin concentrations during extended fasting and graded glucose infusions: relationships with changes in glucose, insulin, and FFA. J Clin Endocrinol Metab 2001;86(10): 4895–900.

111. Wortman MD, Clegg DJ, D'Alessio D, et al. C75 inhibits food intake by increasing CNS glucose metabolism. Nat Med 2003;9(5):483–5.

112. Brownlee M. Biochemistry and molecular cell biology of diabetic complications. Nature 2001;414(6865):813–20.

Central Leucine Sensing in the Control of Energy Homeostasis

Gary J. Schwartz, PhD

KEYWORDS

- Food intake • Leucine • Nutrient sensing • Rapamycin • Diabetes • Obesity
- Hypothalamus • Brainstem

KEY POINTS

- Recent advances identify neuroanatomically distributed nodes in a circuit involving at least two primary leucine sensing sites adjacent to circumventricular organs with preferential access to bloodborne nutrients: the mediobasal hypothalamus and the dorsal vagal complex.
- Activation of these leucine sensing sites engages multiple determinants of energy balance through the mammalian target of rapamycin–S6K and ERK ½ signaling pathways, including glucose homeostasis, food intake, and adiposity.

INTRODUCTION

Leucine is an essential branched chain amino acid (BCAA) that drives intracellular signaling cascades critical to protein synthesis and cellular proliferation via the mammalian target of rapamycin complex 1 (mTORC1)-S6K1 kinase pathway. Both plasma and cerebrospinal leucine levels are rapidly elevated after a high leucine meal[1] and brain access to leucine is mediated by facilitative transport involving both saturable and unsaturable processes.[2] Among amino acid stimuli, l-leucine has been reported to be the most potent activator of p70S6K1.[3] Phosphorylation of S6 kinase, in turn, has been implicated in the negative feedback control of insulin signaling via insulin receptor substrate 1,[4] supporting a potential role for important interactions between leucine and insulin in determining whole body glucose homeostasis through mTORC1-S6K1. In mice, constitutive, systemic deletion of S6K1 protects against diet-induced obesity and enhances insulin sensitivity, yet promotes glucose intolerance.[4] In rats, BCAA supplementation of a high-fat diet (HFD) reduces weight gain while increasing insulin resistance, suggesting that, in the context of HFD, dietary BCAA

Supported by NIH DK 20541 and NIH DK 26687 to GJS.

Department of Medicine, Diabetes Research and Training Center, 1300 Morris Park Avenue, Golding 501, Bronx, NY 10461, USA

E-mail address: gary.schwartz@einstein.yu.edu

Endocrinol Metab Clin N Am 42 (2013) 81–87

http://dx.doi.org/10.1016/j.ecl.2012.12.001

endo.theclinics.com

contributes to the development of insulin resistance during obesity.[5] However, chronic and specific dietary leucine supplementation during HFD has been shown to markedly reduce hyperglycemia, hypercholesteremia, weight gain, and adiposity while increasing resting energy expenditure and molecular activity of uncoupling protein 3 in brown and white adipose tissue, as well as skeletal muscle, without affecting total daily food intake.[6] These apparently disparate findings have driven an ongoing search for specific sites of leucine and downstream p70S6K1 activation important in the control of multiple effectors of energy balance, including glucose homeostasis, food intake, and adiposity. This article reviews results from recent studies identifying two key brain regions as critical nodes in the neural network where central leucine sensing contributes to whole body energy homeostasis. These regions are the mediobasal hypothalamus (MBH, including the arcuate [ARC] and ventromedial [VMH] nuclei) and the dorsal vagal complex of the caudal brainstem (DVC, including the nucleus of the solitary tract [NTS], the dorsal motor vagus, and the area postrema [AP]).

HYPOTHALAMIC LEUCINE AND GLUCOSE HOMEOSTASIS

Important early support for a focus on the central nervous system as a possible site of leucine sensing came from studies of hypothalamic insulin signaling and its role in glucose homeostasis. Results from these studies revealed that central insulin infusions suppressed glucose production during insulin clamp studies in which exogenous glucose is infused to maintain stable glycemia. Central administration of antisense oligonucleotides directed against insulin receptors selectively decreased insulin receptor expression in the MBH and significantly attenuated the ability of central insulin to suppress glucose production during a clamp.[7] Together, these data support an important role for MBH insulin receptors in the ability of central insulin to affect endogenous glucose production. Based on the aforementioned negative feedback relationship between p70S6K1 activation and reduced insulin signaling, Ono and colleagues[8] subsequently investigated the degree to which MBH S6K1 activity might also mediate the ability of hypothalamic insulin to determine glucose homeostasis during a clamp. Acute exposure to HFD elevated hypothalamic S6K1 expression while decreasing central insulin sensitivity. Adenovirally mediated, constitutive activation of S6K1 within the MBH mimicked the ability of HFD to limit central insulin action in the control of glucose production, whereas suppression of hypothalamic S6K1 activity by overexpression of a dominant negative form of the kinase partially reversed the effects of HFD.

Results of these findings supported the possibility that MBH leucine itself, as a potent stimulus of mTOR and S6K1 phosphorylation, would also contribute to the control of glucose homeostasis. Indeed, MBH leucine infusion alone significantly lowered both plasma and glucose levels and, during a basal clamp, MBH leucine suppressed hepatic glucose production by decreasing both glycogenolysis and gluconeogenesis.[9] Pharmacologic or viral blockade of leucine metabolism within the MBH also blocked the ability of MBH leucine to suppress glucose production.[9] Taken together, these data support a specific role for MBH leucine metabolism in the control of glucose homeostasis.

HYPOTHALAMIC LEUCINE AND FOOD INTAKE

Initial studies by Cota and colleagues[10] demonstrated an important role for central leucine and its downstream targets mTOR and S6K1 in the control of food intake and body weight. These studies were advanced by findings that the mTOR-S6K1 pathway was rapidly and robustly activated selectively within MBH ARC neurons expressing anorexigenic pro-opiomelanocortin (POMC) and orexigenic neuropeptide

Y/agouti-related peptide neurons within the ARC during refeeding after a fast. In contrast, hypothalamic paraventricular nucleus (PVN) mTOR and S6K1 activity was unchanged, suggesting that dietary nutrients selectively activated the mTOR-S6K1 pathway within ARC neurons of the MBH. In subsequent studies in fasted rats, the investigators found that third intracerebroventricular (3icv) administration of leucine rapidly stimulated S6K1 activation within the MBH and reduced food intake as early as 4 hours after injection. This reduction persisted for 24 hours, resulting in lower weight gain relative to vehicle-treated controls. Because the MBH is adjacent to the third ventricle site of leucine administration, these data supported the possibility that leucine acted directly on ARC MBH neurons to reduce feeding and body weight gain. In contrast, 3icv administration of l-valine, a non–ketogenic branched chain amino acid used as a control for the chemospecificity of leucine's effects, failed to alter food intake or body weight gain.

The mTOR-S6K1 pathway plays an important role in the ability of 3icv leucine to affect energy intake because coadministration of leucine with subthreshold doses the mTOR inhibitor rapamycin, which had no effect on feeding when administered alone, blocked leucine's effects. Higher doses of rapamycin alone were sufficient to rapidly increase food intake, supporting a role for endogenous leucine sensing in the control of energy balance via mTOR-S6K1.[10] Taken together, these data have been interpreted to support the suggestion that central leucine's feeding suppressive and metabolic effects are mediated by the MBH. However, these studies did not directly challenge this suggestion in two important ways. First, the 3icv administration protocols used did not exclusively target the MBH and, second, there was limited investigation of nonhypothalamic sites, leaving unaddressed the possibility that central leucine sensing at extrahypothalamic sites may also be important in the control of energy balance.

Subsequent studies by Blouet and colleagues addressed both of these concerns, identifying specific roles for MBH leucine and mTOR-S6K1 in the control of energy balance, and revealing the importance of hitherto unreported brainstem leucine sensing capabilities.[1,11] Selective MBH application of l-leucine or equimolar doses of its ketoacid, α-ketoisocaproic acid (KIC), in mice and rats, reduced both short-term feeding, 24 hour cumulative intake, and 24 hour body weight gain, without affecting energy expenditure, locomotor activity, core temperature, or oxygen consumption. In contrast, neither MBH l-valine nor MBH administration of its ketoacid, α-ketoisovaleric acid, had any effect, consistent with the chemospecificity of MBH l-leucine sensing in the hypothalamic control of energy balance. Furthermore, MBH leucine did not support the formation of a conditioned taste aversion. These findings support a feeding specific action of MBH leucine in the control of body weight. Chronic, site-specific pharmacologic inhibition of leucine oxidative metabolism recapitulated the feeding and body weight reductions seen in response to leucine and KIC. The reductions in feeding observed following MBH leucine were due to a selective reduction in meal size, with no acute change in meal frequency, implicating neuronal pathways important in the control of meal size, especially the brainstem, in the feeding suppressive actions of MBH leucine. Taken together, these data: (1) support a role for endogenous leucine metabolism at the MBH in the control of food intake body weight gain and (2) implicate neural substrates important in the control of meal size as likely components of the neural circuitry underlying the behavioral and metabolic effects of MBH leucine sensing.

Results from these studies have also begun to characterize the intracellular and intercellular signaling networks engaged by MBH leucine sensing. Refeeding leucine-rich food after a fast, and MBH leucine itself, each rapidly elevate S6K1 activity selectively within the MBH but not in either PVN or lateral hypothalamic nuclei. These data suggest that MBH leucine's ability to drive S6K1-activation in the MBH may determine leucine's feeding inhibitory actions. Consistent with this suggestion, adeno-virally mediated overexpression of S6K1 within the MBH decreased food intake and reduced body weight gain, and, similar to the effects of MBH leucine, these reductions in feeding were due to a selective reduction in meal size without a change in meal frequency. In contrast, downregulation of S6K1 activity by adenoviral MBH expression of a dominant negative form of the kinase promoted weight gain and increased meal size without increasing meal number.[11]

Refeeding after a fast and MBH leucine administration also activate MBH ERK ½ signaling, implicated in multiple feeding neurocircuits.[12] Pharmacologic ERK ½ inhibition within the MBH rapidly stimulates food intake by selectively increasing meal size. Furthermore, pharmacologic inhibition of ERK ½, at subthreshold doses of ERK antagonists that have no effect when administered alone, are able to block the feeding inhibitory actions on MBH leucine. These data support ERK ½ phosphorylation as an alternative critical signaling mechanism linking MBH leucine sensing to the control of meal size. Biochemical pathways underlying the ability of leucine to drive both S6K1 and ERK phosphorylation remain to be identified.

From an extracellular perspective, MBH leucine induces robust and selective expression of c-fos, a marker of neuronal activation, in multiple forebrain and hindbrain sites, including the ARC, PVN, and the brainstem NTS but not in lateral, supraoptic, or dorsomedial hypothalamic nuclei. Among leucine-activated ARC cells is a population of POMC-expressing neurons, suggesting that leucine sensing stimulates POMC ARC neurons. Consistent with this suggestion, neurophysiological evaluation of hypothalamic slices in vitro revealed that bath application of leucine rapidly stimulated neurophysiological spike activity in identified POMC neurons. MBH leucine also promoted c-fos expression in neurochemically defined oxytocinergic (OXY) neurons within the PVN, supporting an ARC POMC–PVN OXY link, activated by MBH leucine sensing. Because oxytocin has been implicated in the inhibition of food intake, these data raise the possibility that PVN OXY neurons mediate the feeding inhibitory effects of MBH leucine. PVN OXY neurons project, in part, to the caudal brainstem where oxytocin immunoreactive fibers have been localized to the DVC, at the level of the AP, particularly within the NTS. The NTS in this AP-spanning region has been well characterized as a terminus for peripheral neural gastrointestinal meal-related signals important in the negative feedback control of food intake and meal size.[13] Administration of oxytocin receptor antagonists restricted to the fourth ventricle, adjacent to the DVC, robustly and rapidly stimulates food intake and meal size in mice and rats.[14] Furthermore, administration of doses of oxytocin receptor antagonists that had no effect on feeding when administered alone blocked the ability of MBH leucine to reduce meal size.[1] Thus, MBH leucine sensing engages an ARC-PVN-NTS circuit via S6K1, ERK, and oxytocin to control food intake and body weight gain.

BRAINSTEM LEUCINE SENSING IN THE CONTROL OF ENERGY BALANCE

The caudal brainstem DVC is an important site in the neural network engaging multiple effectors of energy balance, including food intake, glucose homeostasis, and thermogenesis. In particular, sensory neurons within the NTS of the DVC mediate the feeding behavioral and metabolic effects of gut nutrient stimulation, gut hormones, the adiposity hormone leptin, and descending hypothalamic inputs from neurons expressing orexigenic and anorexigenic neuropeptides.[15] These neurons are adjacent to the AP, a circumventricular organ with a specialized, fenestrated capillary system that enhances neuronal access to bloodborne factors, presenting the additional possibility of direct nutrient sensing by NTS neurons. This possibility is supported by prior studies indicating that refeeding after a fast rapidly activates not only NTS c-fos expression, but also S6K1 and ERK ½ activation within NTS cells. Consequently, Blouet and Schwartz[16] have recently shown that NTS neurons are directly sensitive to local injections of leucine. In fasted rats primed to eat, direct NTS injections of physiologic doses of leucine rapidly and potently reduced food intake and body weight gain.[16] Within the first several hours postinjection, these reductions in feeding were solely due to reduced meal size and were followed by reductions in both meal size and meal number beginning 6 hours after leucine injection. In contrast, the non–ketogenic amino acid l-valine had no effect on feeding, demonstrating amino acid specificity for leucine nutrient sensing in the NTS, similar to what was found following MBH injection.

NTS leucine also rapidly and potently activated the mTOR pathway, increasing phosphorylation of S6K1 and ribosomal S6 protein, a downstream effector of S6K1. Conversely, direct parenchymal NTS application of the mTOR inhibitor rapamycin stimulated immediate feeding by increasing meal size, supporting a role for endogenous NTS leucine signaling through mTOR-S6K1 in the control of food intake and body weight. Accordingly, NTS application of subthreshold rapamycin doses that had no effect on feeding when administered alone completely blocked the feeding, meal size, and body weight effects of NTS leucine. Furthermore, constitutive adenoviral overexpression of active S6K in the NTS reduced food intake, body weight gain, and adiposity. Also, the reduction in food intake was solely due to smaller meal size, similar to what had been shown following MBH S6K overexpression. These data reveal that there are multiple, parallel, and perhaps redundant roles for leucine sensing in the negative feedback control of food intake, meal size, and body weight, specifically at forebrain and hindbrain regions that abut circumventricular organs.

Immunohistochemical evaluation of the brainstem following NTS leucine injections identified S6K activation in three neurochemically distinct populations: those expressing dopamine beta-hydroxylase, tyrosine hydroxylase, and the anorexigenic peptide precursor POMC. This latter finding suggested that NTS leucine might engage brainstem melanocortin (MC) signaling via POMC NTS neuronal release of melanocortins onto brainstem MC3/4 receptors, implicated in the brainstem control of meal size.[17,18] Consistent with this idea, NTS injection of the MC3/4 antagonist SHU 9119, at doses that had no effect on food intake when administered alone, blocked the ability of NTS leucine to reduce food intake and meal size.

Because the feeding inhibitory effects of brainstem melanocortins are mediated in part by the ERK ½ signaling pathway,[17] subsequent studies evaluated the role of ERK ½ in the ability of brainstem leucine to reduce food intake and meal size. NTS injection of ERK ½ inhibitors alone rapidly increased food intake and meal size, but this effect dissipated within a few hours after antagonist administration without any longer term effect on body weight gain. Furthermore, NTS injections of subthreshold doses of ERK ½ inhibitors, that had no effect on feeding when administered alone, blocked the ability of NTS leucine to reduce food intake and meal size. Thus, NTS leucine sensing mechanisms important in the control of food intake and body weight share several important features in common with MBH leucine sensing: both induce reductions in food intake and body weight gain by selective reductions in meal size, both engage intracellular pathways involving mTOR-S6K and ERK ½ activation, and both seem to be mediated by activation of melanocortinergic signaling.

SUMMARY

Taken together, these recent advances identify neuroanatomically distributed nodes in a circuit involving at least two primary leucine sensing sites adjacent to circumventricular organs, with preferential access to bloodborne nutrients: the MBH and the DVC. Activation of these leucine sensing sites engages multiple determinants of energy balance through the mTOR-S6K and ERK ½ signaling pathways, including glucose homeostasis, food intake, and adiposity. These findings do not exclude the possibility that other important leucine sensing sites may be identified. More importantly, however, the present results raise the question of how these individual, distributed leucine sensing mechanisms act in concert to determine overall energy balance in response to endogenous dietary fluctuations in leucine availability, occurring throughout the cerebral ventricular circulation.

REFERENCES

1. Blouet C, Jo YH, Li X, et al. Mediobasal hypothalamic leucine sensing regulates food intake through activation of a hypothalamus-brainstem circuit. J Neurosci 2009;29:8302–11.
2. Smith QR. The blood-brain barrier and the regulation of amino acid uptake and availability to brain. Adv Exp Med Biol 1991;291:55–71.
3. Shigemitsu K, Tsujishita Y, Miyake H, et al. Structural requirement of leucine for activation of p70 S6 kinase. FEBS Lett 1999;447:303–6.
4. Um SH, Frigerio F, Watanabe M, et al. Absence of S6K1 protects against age- and diet-induced obesity while enhancing insulin sensitivity. Nature 2004;431:200–5.
5. Newgard CB, An J, Bain JR, et al. A branched-chain amino acid-related metabolic signature that differentiates obese and lean humans and contributes to insulin resistance. Cell Metab 2009;9:311–26.
6. Zhang Y, Guo K, LeBlanc RE, et al. Increasing dietary leucine intake reduces diet-induced obesity and improves glucose and cholesterol metabolism in mice via multimechanisms. Diabetes 2007;56:1647–54.
7. Obici S, Feng Z, Karkanias G, et al. Decreasing hypothalamic insulin receptors causes hyperphagia and insulin resistance in rats. Nat Neurosci 2002;5:566–72.
8. Ono H, Pocai A, Wang Y, et al. Activation of hypothalamic S6 kinase mediates diet-induced hepatic insulin resistance in rats. J Clin Invest 2008;118:2959–68.
9. Su Y, Lam TK, He W, et al. Hypothalamic leucine metabolism regulates liver glucose production. Diabetes 2012;61:85–93.
10. Cota D, Proulx K, Smith KA, et al. Hypothalamic mTOR signaling regulates food intake. Science 2006;312:927–30.
11. Blouet C, Ono H, Schwartz GJ. Mediobasal hypothalamic p70 S6 kinase 1 modulates the control of energy homeostasis. Cell Metab 2008;8:459–67.
12. Berthoud HR, Sutton GM, Townsend RL, et al. Brainstem mechanisms integrating gut-derived satiety signals and descending forebrain information in the control of meal size. Physiol Behav 2006;89:517–24.
13. Schwartz GJ. Brainstem integrative function in the central nervous system control of food intake. Forum Nutr 2010;63:141–51.
14. Blevins JE, Schwartz MW, Baskin DG. Evidence that paraventricular nucleus oxytocin neurons link hypothalamic leptin action to caudal brain stem nuclei controlling meal size. Am J Physiol Regul Integr Comp Physiol 2004;287:R87–96.
15. Grill HJ, Hayes MR. Hindbrain neurons as an essential hub in the neuroanatomically distributed control of energy balance. Cell Metab 2012;16:296–309.
16. Blouet C, Schwartz GJ. Brainstem nutrient sensing in the nucleus of the solitary tract inhibits feeding. Cell Metab 2012;16:579–87.

17. Sutton GM, Duos B, Patterson LM, et al. Melanocortinergic modulation of cholecystokinin-induced suppression of feeding through extracellular signal-regulated kinase signaling in rat solitary nucleus. Endocrinology 2005;146:3739–47.
18. Azzara AV, Sokolnicki JP, Schwartz GJ. Central melanocortin receptor agonist reduces spontaneous and scheduled meal size but does not augment duodenal preload-induced feeding inhibition. Physiol Behav 2002;77:411–6.

Novel Aspects of Brown Adipose Tissue Biology

Joerg Heeren, PhD[a],*, Heike Münzberg, PhD[b],*

KEYWORDS

- Brown adipose tissue • Thermogenesis • Neuronal circuits and metabolism
- Lipoprotein metabolism • Triglycerides

KEY POINTS

- Brown adipose tissue (BAT) is existent in human adults; it is able to dissipate excess energy by generating heat, and it might be involved in human body weight control.
- Environmental factors, such as cold, diet, physical activity, and aging, are tightly linked to BAT activity.
- Neuronal and peripheral circuits control BAT-mediated thermogenesis.
- Development of *brownish* adipocytes (so-called beige or brite) in white adipose tissue (WAT) is regulated by diverse factors.
- The activation of BAT and/or browning of WAT are promising targets to treat metabolic diseases, such as diabetes and hyperlipidemia.
- There is an urgent need for prospective studies to unravel the potential use of BAT activation and/or browning for human health.

BROWN ADIPOSE TISSUE AND THERMOREGULATION

In mammals, thermogenesis is necessary to maintain body temperature or generate fevers that fight infection. Thermogenesis also affects energy homeostasis, partially via sympathetic control of brown adipose tissue (BAT) thermogenesis.[1] The importance of BAT thermogenesis in human body weight control has been debated[2,3]; only recently, exciting advances in BAT development have opened new avenues for

Funding sources: Dr Heeren: This work was financially supported by the State Excellence Cluster NAME. Dr Münzberg: This work was financially supported by the National Institute of Health R01-DK092587, P20-RR021945, P30-DK072476.
Conflict of interest: No conflict of interest.
[a] Department of Biochemistry and Molecular Cell Biology, University Medical Center Hamburg-Eppendorf, Martinistraße 52, Hamburg 20246, Germany; [b] Department of Central Leptin Signaling, Pennington Biomedical Research Center, LSU Systems, 6400 Perkins Road, Baton Rouge, LA 70808, USA
* Corresponding author.
E-mail addresses: heeren@uke.de; Heike.Munzberg@pbrc.edu

Endocrinol Metab Clin N Am 42 (2013) 89–107
http://dx.doi.org/10.1016/j.ecl.2012.11.004
0889-8529/13/$ – see front matter © 2013 Elsevier Inc. All rights reserved.

pharmacologic induction of brown adipocytes from progenitor cells within muscle and white adipose tissue.[4] Most importantly, several studies demonstrated substantial amounts of functional BAT in adult humans,[5–8] so that BAT thermogenesis has been rediscovered as a potential target to treat obesity.

Introduction BAT

BAT is a specialized tissue that is able to generate heat and, thus, enables homoiotherm mammals to maintain body temperature largely independent of the environmental temperature. BAT generates heat with the BAT-specific expression of uncoupling protein 1 (UCP1), a proton channel of the inner mitochondrial membrane that allows proton influx into the mitochondrial lumen. The mitochondrial respiratory chain maintains a proton gradient across the inner mitochondrial membrane for ATP production, which is uncoupled by UCP1 to release energy as heat instead.[9–11] This uncoupling process is highly regulated and depends on sympathetic stimulation of β_3-adrenergic receptors (β_3-AR) but is also regulated by fatty acids and thyroid hormone on other stimulants.[12–15] Stimulation of β_3-ARs increases UCP1 gene expression, UCP1 activity, and β-oxidation; β-oxidation is of major importance to fuel the energy-demanding thermogenic process. The induction of BAT thermogenesis is also termed *adaptive thermogenesis* or *nonshivering thermogenesis* to distinguish this highly regulated process from other nonregulated (eg, thermic effects of metabolic processes) or mechanical (eg, shivering) processes that also contribute to heat production.

Induction of BAT Thermogenesis

Exposure to a cold environment robustly stimulates BAT thermogenesis (cold-induced thermogenesis) and is particularly important for small mammals, such as rodents and newborns, because small mammals have a larger surface relative to their body volume compared with large mammals and, thus, lose more heat in a cold environment.[16,17] BAT thermogenesis is also required for normal fever responses (fever-inducing thermogenesis) and is mediated by endogenous pyrogens like prostaglandin E2.[18] It is also well known that the ingestion of food per se as well as caloric-dense diets increases body temperature as well as energy expenditure (diet-induced thermogenesis [DIT]).[19] However, the fact that any meal generally induces energy expenditure and heat production as a mere byproduct of metabolic processes (nonregulated) has elicited some controversial discussions about whether DIT is indeed an adaptive, regulated process or rather an indirect metabolic effect.[2,3]

Controversial Views and Why We Should Mind

In the 70th much effort focused on BAT thermogenesis as an important target for antiobesity drugs and launched intensive studies on DIT in humans. However, the insensitivity of β_3-AR agents in humans, safety issues with drugs that increased BAT thermogenesis (eg, sibutramine),[20] and finally the lack of evidence for substantial amounts of BAT in adult humans led to a cease of research support for DIT-related drug targets. Just recently, a series of publications demonstrated functional and inducible amounts of BAT in at least a subpopulation of adult humans,[5–8] which revived the discussion of adaptive thermogenesis as a potential obesity drug target. Coupled with new insights into the developmental origin of brown adipocytes, central regulation and metabolic dynamics important to induce BAT thermogenesis dramatically highlighted that we were/are still lacking major knowledge about this peculiar heat-generating tissue as well as other potential heat-generating mechanisms in rodents and humans. Thus, there is reasonable hope that continued efforts to understand the role of BAT function in energy homeostasis will boost our approaches to find suitable drug targets to support energy homeostasis control in Western societies.

CENTRAL CONTROL OF BAT THERMOGENESIS
Neuronal Circuits

Much of the recent research has focused on BAT function per se; however, BAT thermogenesis is generally controlled by central mechanisms. Neuroanatomical and pharmacologic approaches based on cold- and pyrogen-induced thermogenesis have identified several central nervous system (CNS) sites as key players in the control of BAT thermogenesis.[21]

Neurons in the hypothalamic preoptic area (POA) act as temperature sensor and integrate temperature information from the CNS, peripheral and deep-body thermoreceptors.[21] POA neurons provide at least inhibitory inputs to the dorsomedial hypothalamus/dorsal hypothalamic area (DMH/DHA).[22–26] Neuronal activation of DMH/DHA neurons, likely representing glutamatergic neurons,[23] is critical for further stimulation of downstream premotor neurons in the rostral raphe pallidus (rRPa)[25,27] to control sympathetic BAT activity (**Fig. 1**). Indeed, typical BAT-inducing stimuli, such as cold, or pyrogens, like lipopolysaccharide (LPS), result in robust stimulation of neuronal activity in rRPa-innervating DMH/DHA neurons.[26,28] The rRPa also receives

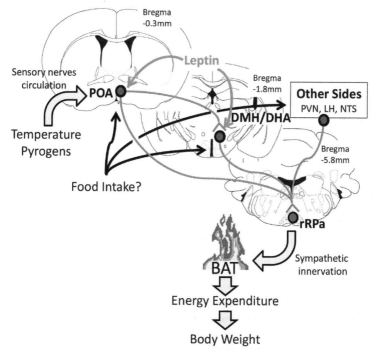

Fig. 1. Central pathways controlling brown fat thermogenesis. Neurons in the POA receive sensory information about ambient temperature (from skin) or pyrogens (from circulation) that is relayed to neurons in the DMH/DHA. Neuronal activation of DMH/DHA neurons stimulates sympathetic premotor neurons in the rostral raphe pallidus to control sympathetic inputs to the BAT. It is still unclear if and where feeding-related signals could integrate into this central thermoregulatory pathway to promote diet-induced thermogenesis. NTS, nucleus of the solitary tract; PVN, paraventricular nucleus located in the hypothalamus; LH, lateral hypothalamus.

direct inputs from the POA[29] and orexin neurons in the lateral hypothalamus[30]; inputs from the nucleus of the solitary tract (NTS) have been hypothesized,[31] even though these circuits have been less well studied.

The ventromedial hypothalamus (VMH) had been historically associated with thermoregulatory control[32–34]; but recent work suggested that the anatomically large size of deletions and injections may have confounded the original conclusions, and the observed thermogenic effects could have resulted from leakage into the nearby DMH/DHA structure.[27,35] Indeed, the DMH/DHA has been well demonstrated to play a crucial role in the regulation of BAT thermogenesis and responds to thermoregulatory drugs more sensitively than the VMH.[36] However, the DMH is also known for its exceptional interconnection with virtually all other hypothalamic sites, including the VMH,[37] so that it is still possible that VMH neurons regulate thermoregulation indirectly through innervation of the DMH/DHA.

Sensing Processes for BAT Thermogenesis: from Cold and Pyrogens to Ingested Diets

Thermoregulatory control is initiated via sensory neurons in the skin, abdomen, and spinal cord but also via thermosensing neurons in the CNS (eg, warm-sensing neurons in the POA).[38] Fever responses to LPS can be initiated by prostaglandin receptor (PGE$_2$)–expressing POA neurons[39] that also regulate BAT thermogenesis via the DMH/DHA and rRPa neurons.[26] However, very little is known about the sensory systems that could connect changes in dietary content with thermoregulatory control mechanisms (diet-induced thermogenesis); it is not entirely clear if cold- and diet-induced thermogenesis are indeed regulated by identical systems.

Temperature-sensing mechanisms have been studied in POA neurons whereby warm- and cold-sensing neurons can be distinguished because of increased firing rates with hypothalamic warming or cooling, respectively.[40–42] There is strong evidence that neuronal cold sensitivity is caused by (GABAergic) synaptic inhibition from warm-sensing neurons.[40,43–46] DMH/DHA neurons have characteristics similar to these cold-sensing neurons because cold exposure increases their activity[25–27,47,48] and they are inhibited by GABAergic inputs at least from the POA.[22,25,26,47,49–51] Neuronal coupling with other sensory systems that also influence body temperature control (eg, neurons regulated by glucose, fasting, or reproductive hormones) may further influence neuronal firing and transmitter release within these systems, even though this has not been investigated yet.

The Melanocortin System, Thermoregulation, and Energy Expenditure

The hypothalamic arcuate nucleus senses and reacts to changes in feeding states (eg, high-fat diet or fasting). Particularly, the melanocortin system consists of anorexigenic pro-opiomelanocortin (POMC) neurons and orexigenic agouti-related-peptide (AgRP) neurons that are differentially regulated in response to feeding states.[52] POMC and AgRP neurons both project broadly within the hypothalamus, including the POA and DMH.[53] Indeed, melanocortin-4-receptors (MC4R) are found in many neurons associated with the regulation of sympathetic BAT inputs[54]; MC4R function in cholinergic intermediolateral nucleus neurons is sufficient to recover the low-energy expenditure of MC4R-deficient mice.[55] Intriguingly, MC4R-deficient mice are very prone to gain weight but fail to raise UCP1 in response to a high fat diet (HFD),[54,56] indicating that MC4R signaling is an important component to induce diet-induced thermogenesis. Thus, the melanocortin system would be well positioned to serve as a sensory relay between the feeding state and thermoregulatory control in diet-induced obesity.

The Leptin System Thermoregulation and Energy Expenditure

Leptin is an adipocyte-derived hormone that is well known to mediate its anorexigenic effects via the melanocortin system. However, targeted deletion of leptin receptors (LepRb) from AgRP and/or POMC neurons did not substantially modulate energy expenditure.[57,58] In contrast, the complete lack of leptin signaling results in hypothermia, cold sensitivity,[59–62] BAT atrophy, and decreased UCP1 expression,[63,64] clearly demonstrating an important function of leptin in thermoregulatory control. Leptin mediates food-independent body weight loss[65] that depends on UCP1 expression,[66] suggesting that food-independent body weight control by leptin is mediated via BAT thermogenesis. Also, fat oxidation (a key thermoregulatory function to fuel mitochondrial respiration) is centrally controlled by leptin via AMP-kinase (AMPK) pathways.[67–69] Similarly, in humans, leptin prevents decreased energy expenditure commonly associated with dieting,[70] even though it remains unclear if this involves central mechanisms or regulation of peripheral tissues (eg, BAT, muscle) to increase energy expenditure.

LepRb are expressed in the POA and DMH/DHA, and these LepRb neurons recapitulate known thermoregulatory circuits; POA and DMH/DHA LepRb neurons are associated with sympathetic BAT innervation and both innervate the rRPa. POA LepRb neurons innervate the DMH/DHA, and DMH/DHA LepRb neurons are robustly stimulated by cold exposure,[71] indicating that leptin uses identical circuits as cold or pyrogens to regulate thermogenesis. The effect of leptin on energy expenditure and body temperature is most robust in states of low leptin levels (eg, leptin deficiency and fasting), and it has been argued that leptin has a rather permissive than actively thermogenic effect. However, other studies also confirm in normal-fed rodents that leptin effectively increases sympathetic BAT activity, BAT temperature, and body core temperature.[72–74] Furthermore, high-fat-diet–induced hyperleptinemia is further associated with increased body temperature, indicating that leptin, in fact, contributes to the induction of diet-induced thermogenesis.[72] Thus, the capacity of this thermoregulatory leptin system to regulate energy expenditure and body weight remains to be tested. Also, the cellular mechanisms involved to regulate neuronal activity (eg, in DMH/DHA LepRb neurons by cold exposure and supposedly by leptin) are unknown.

Thermoregulatory leptin action can also be mediated by brainstem mechanisms independent of hypothalamic function, as observed in decerebrated rats.[75] Although fourth ventricle leptin alone only mildly raises body or brown fat temperature, leptin robustly enhanced thermogenic capacities of thyroid-releasing hormone (TRH).[31,76] This sensitizing effect was dependent on phospholipase C and inositol-3-phosphate calcium release mechanisms and could be attributed to direct leptin effects on NTS neurons.[77] These NTS neurons may further stimulate rRPa neurons to control BAT thermogenesis, even though these connections remain to be validated.

Other Central Regulators of Thermogenesis and Energy Expenditure

Central thyroid function and AMPK signaling

Thyroid hormone is well known to regulate body temperature and energy expenditure via its function in peripheral organs.[14] Thyroxin (T4) is the predominant form of thyroid hormone in the circulation and is converted to the more potent form triiodothyronine (T3) by deiodinases in local target tissues like BAT and white adipose tissue, liver, and muscle. Such deiodinases are also found in the brain indicating that thyroid hormone may also regulate metabolic function via central mechanisms.[78] This finding has been further confirmed by hypothalamic T3 injections, which increases energy expenditure and body temperature via inactivation of AMPK signaling pathways and further activated rRPa neurons.[79] Thus, thyroid hormone may also regulate these typical cold- and pyrogen-induced thermoregulatory circuits.

Leptin also deactivates hypothalamic AMPK signaling, which is well known to modulate feeding behavior, in part via regulation of POMC and AgRP expression[67]; and it is possible that thermogenic leptin actions are also mediated via hypothalamic AMPK pathways. Also, bone morphogenetic protein 8B (BMP8B) importantly regulates energy expenditure and body temperature via central mechanisms that involve AMPK signaling and ultimately results in neuronal activation of rRPa neurons.[80] However, it remains unclear which cellular mechanisms are regulated by hypothalamic AMPK that would explain neuronal excitation in brainstem rRPa neurons.

In peripheral tissues, AMPK is known as a master energy sensor and regulator of lipid metabolism. AMPK is upregulated by increased ATP demand (thus high AMP/ATP ratio), and activation of AMPK enables enhanced β-oxidation and free fatty acid (FFA) transport to fuel mitochondrial energy generation.[81] In the brain, AMPK is inversely regulated to the periphery, but how this relates to cellular processes within the brain (eg, changes in lipid metabolism, gene expression, neuronal activity) is not well understood and requires further investigations.

Thermoregulatory neuropeptide Y action in the dorsomedial hypothalamus

The DMH harbors a well-described population of neurons that expresses thermoregulatory neuropeptide Y (NPY), which is greatly enhanced in states of increased energy demand[82,83] or in rodent models of obesity.[84–87] Viral knockdown of NPY mRNA selectively in the DMH increased UCP1 expression in BAT as well as white fat, which resulted in increased energy expenditure.[88] This effect was mediated via sympathetic innervation of at least the white fat, even though whether NPY neurons feed into the thermoregulatory circuit (POA > DMH/DHA > rRPa) remains to be tested.

PERIPHERAL CONTROL OF BAT THERMOGENESIS
Cell Types Responsible for Thermogenesis: the Origin of Brown and Beige (Brite) Adipocytes

There are multiple fat depots all over the body containing different cell types important for energy storage and thermogenesis.[89] Excess energy is stored in white adipocytes in one large lipid droplet, whereas brown adipocytes realize the combination of lipid storage in multilocular lipid droplets and energy combustion by abundant mitochondria. Classical brown adipocytes, located, for instance, in the interscapular region of mice, share a developmental Myf5-positive precursor with muscle cells.[90] Critically involved in brown adipocyte commitment and differentiation are nuclear receptors, such as peroxisome proliferator activated receptors (PPARs), and their respective transcriptional coactivators, such as PGC1α and PRDM16 (for review see[91]). Thermogenic stimuli also induce the appearance of UCP1-expressing brownlike fat cells, especially in subcutaneous white adipose tissue depots. These beige or brite (made up of brown in white) adipocytes arise from discrete progenitor cells in white adipose tissue[92,93] in a process that is again dependent on the expression of PGC1α and PRDM16.[94] Browning is regulated by several signals, including central and endocrine signals, which are discussed in more detail later. Recently, it was demonstrated that human brown adipose tissue resembled more closely those of murine beige adipocytes than of classical brown adipocytes, at least when comparing gene expression signatures from human brown adipose tissue with fat depots taken from mice.[95] However, it should be emphasized that although the development of these UCP1-positive adipocytes is associated with beneficial effects on body weight and metabolic health,[94] it is still unclear whether beige adipocytes arising in white adipose tissue of mice are as powerful as their classical brown adipocyte relatives.

Hormones Controlling BAT Development and Function

The development of brown and beige adipocytes is regulated by diverse factors in an endocrine, paracrine, and autocrine fashion (**Fig. 2**). Next to catecholamines, the pleiotropic role of thyroid hormones, sex hormones, bile acids, endocannabinoids, and corticosteroids for BAT biology has been summarized in several excellent reviews.[1,96–98] Recent reports indicate that also prostaglandins, members of the fibroblast growth factor (FGF) family, BMP, cardiac natriuretic peptides, and a novel myokine called irisin are important peripheral modulators for BAT development and thermogenesis.

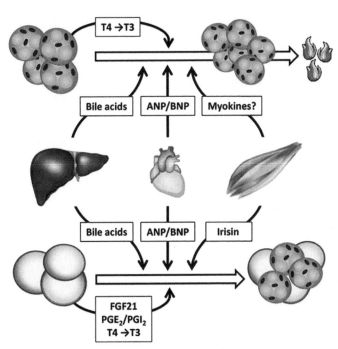

Fig. 2. Peripheral signals controlling brown and brite adipose tissue. Next to activation via the sympathetic nervous system, diverse endocrine signals, such as bile acids or natriuretic peptides (atrial natriuretic peptides [ATP] and brain natriuretic peptides [BNP]), increase energy expenditure by the induction of thermogenic genes in BAT. These hepatocyte- and cardiomyocyte-specific factors also positively influence the development of UCP1-expressing, multilocular so-called beige or brite adipocytes, which are characterized by an intermediate phenotype between brown and white adipocytes. Irisin, a myokine released by exercised muscles, stimulates only specific precursor cells within the white but not the BAT to develop a brownish phenotype. Next to endocrine control, specific prostaglandins and fibroblast growth factor 21 (FGF21) released by white adipocytes initiate the browning in an autocrine and/or paracrine manner. In addition, the 2-mediated conversion of thyroxine (T4) into triiodothyronine (T3) further promotes activation and development of brown and brite adipocytes, respectively. Both the activation of BAT but also the occurrence of brite adipose tissue is associated with a beneficial metabolic profile, implying that both processes are important for the maintenance of metabolic health.

Prostaglandins

The generation of fatty acid–derived prostaglandins is controlled by 2 cyclooxygenase isoenzymes (COX1 and COX2). The latter is induced by β-adrenergic signaling after long-term cold exposure in white adipose tissue, which is associated with an increase in PGE_2/PGI_2 levels. Interestingly, selective COX2 overexpression in white adipose tissue leads to de novo recruitment of beige adipocytes, thereby preventing high-fat-diet–induced obesity by increased energy expenditure.[99] Accordingly, cold-induced UCP1 expression is attenuated in white adipose tissue of COX2-deficient mice,[100] underlining that the manipulation of this novel signaling pathway might be an alternative strategy to induce slimming by browning.[101]

FGFs

There are several FGF family members that have been implicated in the regulation of adipose tissue function. Autocrine and/or paracrine signaling are mediated via the interaction of FGFs with their respective FGF receptors and heparin.[102] The prototype of this protein family, FGF1, is increased in obesity and seems to be the main functional FGF protein, at least in human subcutaneous white adipose tissue.[103] In line with this observation, as a direct target of the adipose tissue master regulator PPARγ, FGF1 is a critical transducer of environmental signals to maintain white adipose tissue function.[104]

Members of the FGF19 subfamily, including FGF21, can also exert endocrine functions by activating FGF receptors complexed to klotho proteins.[105] In mice, FGF21 expression is induced by treatment with PPARα agonist and fasting in liver, by treatment with PPARγ agonist and feeding in white adipose tissue, or by cold exposure in brown adipocytes.[106,107] Because circulating plasma levels of FGF21 corresponds to its hepatic expression, the endocrine function, such as the induction of fat oxidation in response to fasting, is mediated exclusively by liver-derived FGF21. However, antidiabetic properties of PPARγ agonist seems to be dependent on FGF21 synthesized in white adipose tissue. Mechanistically, FGF21 prevents PPARγ inactivation by inhibiting its conversion to an inactive, sumoylated form of PPARγ.[106] In addition, by enhancing PGC1α protein levels, FGF21 is also critical for the development of beige adipocytes. Consequently, FGF21 deficiency is associated with decreased browning and an impaired adaptation to cold exposure.[108] In summary, over the past years, FGF21 has evolved as a strong metabolic regulator, positively influencing energy expenditure probably via inducing the development of beige adipocytes. However, to gain a more comprehensive picture of FGF21 biology in humans and to decipher its potential adverse effects on skeleton,[109] future work will have to elucidate its suitability to treat metabolic diseases in clinical studies.

BMPs

BMPs are secreted molecules that are known to induce the differentiation of mesenchymal toward bone-forming cells, the osteoblast.[110] BMP7-mediated signaling induces not only the key transcription factor for osteoblast differentiation, RUNX2,[111] but also promotes differentiation of brown preadipocytes leading to the induction of PRDM16 and PGC1α. Consequently, the lack of BMP7 results in an almost complete absence of UCP1, whereas BMP7 overexpression increases brown adipose tissue mass and energy expenditure.[112] As described earlier,(see "Other Central Regulators of Thermogenesis and Energy Expenditure" section), another BMP family member, BMP8B, is involved in the regulation of hypothalamic AMPK activity.[80] In addition, BMP8B expression is also induced in mature brown adipocytes in response to thermogenic stimuli, such as diet and cold exposure, thereby enhancing noradrenaline-mediated signaling via stimulation of P38-MAPK and phosphorylation of the cAMP response element-binding protein (CREB).[80] Consequently, BMP8B-deficient mice display an obesogenic phenotype probably mediated by both central and peripheral actions.

Cardiac Natriuretic Peptides

Atrial and brain natriuretic peptides (ANP and BNP, respectively) are produced in the heart to maintain the homeostasis of body fluids and blood pressure. It is well established that cold exposure raises blood pressure, thereby triggering cardiovascular complications in winter.[113] Thus, the release of cardiac hormones to activate thermogenesis for heat production would make physiologic sense to prevent cold-induced hypertension. Natriuretic peptides can bind to their respective receptors present on adipocytes to stimulate lipolysis via cGMP-dependent signaling,[114] a pathway also known to control brown fat cell differentiation and mitochondrial biogenesis.[115] Recently, Bordicchia and colleagues[116] described that increased levels of both ANP and BNP as a consequence of cold exposure or infusion of recombinant proteins leads to the expression of PGC1α and UCP1 in white and brown adipose tissue. This intriguing report clearly demonstrates that cardiac hormones are peripheral regulators for heat production, a process that might, from an evolutionary perspective, be developed to counteract cold-induced harmful effects, such as cardiac hypertrophy and hypertension.

Muscle-Derived Irisin

Similarly, to the adaptive response of the heart, skeletal muscle should also activate energy expenditure by adipose tissue to circumvent the detrimental effects of shivering thermogenesis. Boström and colleagues[117] showed that this concept might indeed have evolved since exercised muscle cells increase the expression of FNDC5. After proteolytic cleavage by an unknown shedding enzyme, this membrane protein is released into the circulation as a hormone called irisin, a myokine driving beige adipocyte development within white adipose tissue. Despite the attractive hypothesis that beneficial metabolic effects of exercise are in part explained by the browning of white adipose tissue, open questions, including the molecular targets of irisin responsible for beige adipocyte differentiation as well as the relevance of irisin for human physiology, remain to be solved.

BAT-MEDIATED REGULATION OF FUEL DELIVERY
BAT as a New Player in Lipoprotein Metabolism

Cold exposure results in the acute breakdown of cellular triglyceride stores within brown adipocytes, which are used as fuel for heat production.[1] To sustain their function, brown adipocytes rely on supply with glucose and fatty acids. In fact, up to 90% of energy for heat production is derived from fatty acids, which are the main source for β-oxidation in brown adipocytes.[1] Fatty acids are mainly transported as esterified triglycerides by 2 classes of lipoproteins that are responsible for the transport of energy to the different organs via the circulation; chylomicrons are formed in the intestine to deliver dietary fat in the postprandial phase, whereas very low-density lipoprotein are produced in the liver when food supply is low. In the bloodstream, these triglyceride-rich lipoproteins (TRL) are hydrolyzed by lipoprotein lipase (LPL), which results in the release of nonesterified fatty acids (NEFAs) and their subsequent internalization by fatty acid transporters into muscle or adipose tissues. LPL activity is controlled by several proteins, including apolipoproteins and angiopoietinlike proteins (reviewed by[118,119]), ensuring that energy is transported into the right tissue dependent on the metabolic conditions. Thus, the regulation of LPL activity fulfills an important gatekeeper function for energy delivery to metabolically active tissues. In addition, LPL is able to facilitate the interaction with lipoprotein receptors to enhance lipoprotein clearance.[120] In activated BAT, local LPL activity is enormously induced ensuring fatty acid uptake as a fuel for heat production. Recent work from the authors' group demonstrated that the triglyceride-lowering effect of LPL in stimulated BAT is mediated in concert with the fatty acid transporter CD36.[121] In addition to NEFAs, whole TRL particles were internalized in an LPL-dependent manner at the vascular endothelium into brown adipocytes. Given that the liver is equipped with a fenestrated endothelium enabling direct contact with plasma lipoproteins, TRL particle uptake into BAT either involves leakage of the endothelial layer or requires transendothelial transport. This study strongly implicates that lipids are, to a large extent, transported by lipoproteins to brown adipocytes. However, the biologic importance and the underlying mechanisms of lipoprotein uptake into BAT is still unclear, but it seems that these processes are fundamentally different from canonical lipoprotein pathways found in skeletal muscle or white adipose tissue.[121–124]

BAT Function: Regulated by Fatty Acids?

Fatty acids not only serve as fuels but they can also act as ligands for transcription factors of the PPAR family.[125] For instance, NEFAs released from intracellular triglyceride stores by adipose triglyceride lipase have been shown to promote PPARα function in the heart.[126] The molecular program initiated in response to cold in BAT is induced by PPARα, PPARγ, PGC1α, as well as the aforementioned PRDM16.[127,128] In this light, lipoprotein-mediated delivery of lipids to brown adipocytes could be directly linked to mitochondrial activity and energy expenditure through the PPAR-activating properties of certain triglyceride lipolysis products. Given that 50% of a lipid-rich meal end up in BAT when mice are exposed to cold,[129] it is a conceivable and intriguing concept that diets, especially the composition of ingested fatty acids, could directly influence the thermogenic program of BAT.

BAT THERMOGENESIS AND BODY WEIGHT CONTROL
Mouse Models

There is no doubt that BAT thermogenesis is the key tissue to maintain homeothermy in small mammals and newborns in cold environments. This point has been greatly confirmed in mice with genetic deletion of UCP1 (UCP1-knockout [KO] mice), which are unable to survive acute cold exposure.[130] BAT thermogenesis is obviously a very energy-demanding process and impacts whole-body energy homeostasis as demonstrated by the robust increase in food intake observed during cold exposure, while body weight is maintained. Thus, it was expected that UCP1-KO mice would develop obesity. Surprisingly, UCP1-KO mice were leaner than their wild-type littermates,[130] strongly arguing against a role of BAT thermogenesis for body weight control. In contrast, when put on a high-fat diet under thermoneutral conditions (eliminating the need for compensatory thermogenic mechanisms that could override the UCP1 deficiency phenotype[131]), UCP1-KO mice indeed gain more weight than control littermates,[132] even though this was not found by others.[130] Furthermore, overexpression of UCP1 in epididymal fat tissue resulted in a marked metabolic improvement beyond the expected heat-generating UCP1 function. Indeed, mild UPC1 overexpression that did not cause a change in energy expenditure resulted in a robust leptin and insulin sensitizing effect and involved afferent nerve signals from fat to the brain.[133] Thus, although the previously described mouse models convincingly connect BAT thermogenesis with body weight loss, there still remains some debate if this can be solely explained by typical heat-generating UCP1 mechanisms.

Yet, the main question remains regarding how BAT thermogenesis can be safely modulated without severe side effects (eg, cardiac dysfunction), which will require a better understanding of central and peripheral regulators of BAT thermogenesis. Although the central pathways regulating sympathetic BAT inputs have been well defined, it is not clear if these circuits also control other peripheral tissues (eg, white fat, liver, skeletal, or heart muscle). Similarly, novel hormones like irisin may not be restricted to peripheral actions but could also engage central circuits to regulate thermogenic function.

Humans

To visualize the metabolism of cancer cells, noninvasive metabolic imaging has been established with radiolabeled substrates, such as ^{18}F-desoxyglucose in nuclear imaging modalities, like positron emission tomography (PET). The combination of PET with computed tomography (PET/CT) allows determining the exact localization of glucose uptake. BAT was long thought to be only of relevance in children and small mammals; but by using this PET/CT technology to reevaluate ^{18}F-desoxyglucose uptake patterns, high metabolic activity was found within the fatty tissue of shoulders, neck, and thoracic spine, especially in underweight patients. Although it was not proven at that time, the investigators proposed that these depots could represent activated brown adipose tissue.[134] Meanwhile, it is accepted that the prevalence of functional BAT ranges from 30% to 100% depending on the respective cohort analyzed (for review see[135,136]) and that BAT activity declines in obese and elderly people.[5,135,137,138] However, in comparison with mice, the amount of active BAT in humans is approximately 100-fold lower,[122,139] arguing against a significant role of human BAT for energy metabolism. Nevertheless, dedicated studies imply that selective drugs sustaining or increasing BAT activity might have beneficial effects on obesity and metabolic health. For example, based on PET/CT tracer studies, Virtanen and colleagues[138] calculated the weight of supraclavicular BAT depots for one individual with 63 g, which, if fully activated, would be able to dissipate an energy equivalent of approximately 4.1 kg during 1 year. Characteristic metabolic alterations that commonly accompany obesity and diabetes are low levels of high-density lipoproteins (HDL) and increased plasma triglycerides. Notably, LPL and brown fatlike gene expression patterns in epicardial adipose tissue correlate positively with HDL cholesterol and negatively with plasma triglyceride levels in patients who are dyslipidemic,[140] suggesting that BAT activation improve plasma lipoprotein profile not only in rodents. This intriguing concept of induced energy expenditure mediated by BAT as a promising strategy to facilitate weight loss received further support by a very elegant study using different radiolabeled tracers.[141] The investigators showed that BAT activated by acute cold exposure significantly contributes to oxidative metabolism and fuel uptake in humans, emphasizing the potential of BAT as an energy sink to lose weight. In addition, Orava and colleagues[142] showed in cold-exposed healthy individuals a positive association between whole-body energy expenditure and BAT perfusion. Interestingly and in contrast to rodents, cold exposure but not sympathomimetic ephedrine activates human BAT,[143] accentuating the need to determine molecular targets and pathways in central and peripheral organs that are activated by cold exposure in humans.

SUMMARY AND OUTLOOK

During the last decades, obesity research has focused on food intake regulation, whereas energy expenditure has been mainly measured based on whole-body oxygen consumption. With the renaissance of BAT thermogenesis as a potential drug target in humans, more thought is put into alternative heat-producing mechanisms. Also, the interaction of peripheral and central components to regulate thermogenesis requires further studies, including central control of sympathetic outputs, humoral control of fat browning, and the importance of BAT activity to controlled lipid homeostasis. Certainly, several of the novel molecular genetic tools available now, compared with 40 years ago, will be helpful to gain new insights in BAT-controlled energy homeostasis and promises new approaches to pharmacologically control body weight.

REFERENCES

1. Cannon B, Nedergaard J. Brown adipose tissue: function and physiological significance. Physiol Rev 2004;84:277–359.
2. Kozak LP. Brown fat and the myth of diet-induced thermogenesis. Cell Metab 2010;11:263–7.
3. Cannon B, Nedergaard J. Nonshivering thermogenesis and its adequate measurement in metabolic studies. J Exp Biol 2011;214:242–53.
4. Seale P, Kajimura S, Spiegelman BM. Transcriptional control of brown adipocyte development and physiological function–of mice and men. Genes Dev 2009;23: 788–97.
5. van Marken Lichtenbelt WD, Vanhommerig JW, Smulders NM, et al. Cold-activated brown adipose tissue in healthy men. N Engl J Med 2009;360:1500–8.
6. Ravussin E, Kozak LP. Have we entered the brown adipose tissue renaissance? Obes Rev 2009;10:265–8.
7. Fruhbeck G, Becerril S, Sainz N, et al. BAT: a new target for human obesity? Trends Pharmacol Sci 2009;30:387–96.
8. Nedergaard J, Bengtsson T, Cannon B. Unexpected evidence for active brown adipose tissue in adult humans. Am J Physiol Endocrinol Metab 2007;293:E444–52.
9. Aquila H, Link TA, Klingenberg M. The uncoupling protein from brown fat mitochondria is related to the mitochondrial ADP/ATP carrier. Analysis of sequence homologies and of folding of the protein in the membrane. EMBO J 1985;4:2369–76.
10. Heaton GM, Wagenvoord RJ, Kemp A Jr, et al. Brown-adipose-tissue mitochondria: photoaffinity labelling of the regulatory site of energy dissipation. Eur J Biochem 1978;82:515–21.
11. Nicholls DG, Rial E. A history of the first uncoupling protein, UCP1. J Bioenerg Biomembr 1999;31:399–406.
12. Himms-Hagen J, Cui J, Danforth E Jr, et al. Effect of CL-316,243, a thermogenic beta 3-agonist, on energy balance and brown and white adipose tissues in rats. Am J Physiol 1994;266:R1371–82.
13. Bartness TJ, Vaughan CH, Song CK. Sympathetic and sensory innervation of brown adipose tissue. Int J Obes (Lond) 2010;34(Suppl 1):S36–42.
14. Silva JE. Thermogenic mechanisms and their hormonal regulation. Physiol Rev 2006;86:435–64.
15. Prusiner SB, Cannon B, Lindberg O. Oxidative metabolism in cells isolated from brown adipose tissue. 1. Catecholamine and fatty acid stimulation of respiration. Eur J Biochem 1968;6:15–22.
16. Heldmaier G, Klaus S, Wiesinger H, et al. Cold acclimation and thermogenesis. In: Malan A, Canguilhem B, editors. "Living in the cold" 2nd International Symposium, 1989.
17. Griggio MA. Thermogenic mechanisms in cold-acclimated animals. Braz J Med Biol Res 1988;21:171–6.

18. Elmquist JK, Scammell TE, Saper CB. Mechanisms of CNS response to systemic immune challenge: the febrile response. Trends Neurosci 1997;20:565–70.
19. Rothwell NJ, Stock MJ. A role for brown adipose tissue in diet-induced thermogenesis. Nature 1979;281:31–5.
20. Clapham JC, Arch JR. Targeting thermogenesis and related pathways in anti-obesity drug discovery. Pharmacol Ther 2011;131:295–308.
21. Morrison SF, Nakamura K, Madden CJ. Central control of thermogenesis in mammals. Exp Physiol 2008;93:773–97.
22. Nakamura K, Matsumura K, Kaneko T, et al. The rostral raphe pallidus nucleus mediates pyrogenic transmission from the preoptic area. J Neurosci 2002;22:4600–10.
23. Cao WH, Morrison SF. Glutamate receptors in the raphe pallidus mediate brown adipose tissue thermogenesis evoked by activation of dorsomedial hypothalamic neurons. Neuropharmacology 2006;51:426–37.
24. Cao WH, Fan W, Morrison SF. Medullary pathways mediating specific sympathetic responses to activation of dorsomedial hypothalamus. Neuroscience 2004;126:229–40.
25. Nakamura Y, Nakamura K, Matsumura K, et al. Direct pyrogenic input from prostaglandin EP3 receptor-expressing preoptic neurons to the dorsomedial hypothalamus. Eur J Neurosci 2005;22:3137–46.
26. Yoshida K, Li X, Cano G, et al. Parallel preoptic pathways for thermoregulation. J Neurosci 2009;29:11954–64.
27. Dimicco JA, Zaretsky DV. The dorsomedial hypothalamus: a new player in thermoregulation. Am J Physiol Regul Integr Comp Physiol 2007;292:R47–63.
28. Sarkar S, Zaretskaia MV, Zaretsky DV, et al. Stress- and lipopolysaccharide-induced c-fos expression and nNOS in hypothalamic neurons projecting to medullary raphe in rats: a triple immunofluorescent labeling study. Eur J Neurosci 2007;26:2228–38.
29. Hermann DM, Luppi PH, Peyron C, et al. Afferent projections to the rat nuclei raphe magnus, raphe pallidus and reticularis gigantocellularis pars alpha demonstrated by iontophoretic application of choleratoxin (subunit b). J Chem Neuroanat 1997;13:1–21.
30. Tupone D, Madden CJ, Cano G, et al. An orexinergic projection from perifornical hypothalamus to raphe pallidus increases rat brown adipose tissue thermogenesis. J Neurosci 2011;31:15944–55.
31. Rogers RC, Barnes MJ, Hermann GE. Leptin "gates" thermogenic action of thyrotropin-releasing hormone in the hindbrain. Brain Res 2009;1295:135–41.
32. Yoshida T, Bray GA. Catecholamine turnover in rats with ventromedial hypothalamic lesions. Am J Physiol 1984;246:R558–65.
33. Perkins MN, Rothwell NJ, Stock MJ, et al. Activation of brown adipose tissue thermogenesis by the ventromedial hypothalamus. Nature 1981;289:401–2.
34. Kelly L, Bielajew C. Ventromedial hypothalamic regulation of brown adipose tissue. Neuroreport 1991;2:41–4.
35. Dimicco JA, Samuels BC, Zaretskaia MV, et al. The dorsomedial hypothalamus and the response to stress: part renaissance, part revolution. Pharmacol Biochem Behav 2002;71:469–80.
36. Samuels BC, Zaretsky DV, Dimicco JA. Dorsomedial hypothalamic sites where disinhibition evokes tachycardia correlate with location of raphe-projecting neurons. Am J Physiol Regul Integr Comp Physiol 2004;287:R472–8.
37. Ter Horst GJ, Luiten PG. The projections of the dorsomedial hypothalamic nucleus in the rat. Brain Res Bull 1986;16:231–48.

38. Morrison SF, Madden CJ, Tupone D. Central control of brown adipose tissue thermogenesis. Front Endocrinol (Lausanne) 2012;3. pii: 00005.
39. Lazarus M, Yoshida K, Coppari R, et al. EP3 prostaglandin receptors in the median preoptic nucleus are critical for fever responses. Nat Neurosci 2007;10:1131–3.
40. Boulant JA. Neuronal basis of Hammel's model for set-point thermoregulation. J Appl Physiol 2006;100:1347–54.
41. Griffin JD, Boulant JA. Temperature effects on membrane potential and input resistance in rat hypothalamic neurones. J Physiol 1995;488(Pt 2):407–18.
42. Griffin JD, Kaple ML, Chow AR, et al. Cellular mechanisms for neuronal thermosensitivity in the rat hypothalamus. J Physiol 1996;492(Pt 1):231–42.
43. Kelso SR, Boulant JA. Effect of synaptic blockade on thermosensitive neurons in hypothalamic tissue slices. Am J Physiol 1982;243:R480–90.
44. Fregly MJ, Blatteis CM, editors. Handbook of physiology. Section 4: Environmental Physiology. Volume 1. New York: Oxford University Press; 1996. p. 105–26.
45. Dean JB, Boulant JA. Effects of synaptic blockade on thermosensitive neurons in rat diencephalon in vitro. Am J Physiol 1989;257:R65–73.
46. Kelso SR, Perlmutter MN, Boulant JA. Thermosensitive single-unit activity of in vitro hypothalamic slices. Am J Physiol 1982;242:R77–84.
47. Cano G, Passerin AM, Schiltz JC, et al. Anatomical substrates for the central control of sympathetic outflow to interscapular adipose tissue during cold exposure. J Comp Neurol 2003;460:303–26.
48. Boulant JA, Chow AR, Griffin JD. Determinants of hypothalamic neuronal thermosensitivity. Ann N Y Acad Sci 1997;813:133–8.
49. Hunt JL, Zaretsky DV, Sarkar S, et al. Dorsomedial hypothalamus mediates autonomic, neuroendocrine, and locomotor responses evoked from the medial preoptic area. Am J Physiol Regul Integr Comp Physiol 2010;298:R130–40.
50. Zaretskaia MV, Zaretsky DV, Sarkar S, et al. Induction of Fos-immunoreactivity in the rat brain following disinhibition of the dorsomedial hypothalamus. Brain Res 2008;1200:39–50.
51. Zaretskaia MV, Zaretsky DV, Dimicco JA. Role of the dorsomedial hypothalamus in thermogenesis and tachycardia caused by microinjection of prostaglandin E2 into the preoptic area in anesthetized rats. Neurosci Lett 2003;340:1–4.
52. Schwartz MW, Woods SC, Porte D Jr, et al. Central nervous system control of food intake. Nature 2000;404:661–71.
53. Bagnol D, Lu XY, Kaelin CB, et al. Anatomy of an endogenous antagonist: relationship between Agouti-related protein and proopiomelanocortin in brain. J Neurosci 1999;19:RC26.
54. Voss-Andreae A, Murphy JG, Ellacott KL, et al. Role of the central melanocortin circuitry in adaptive thermogenesis of brown adipose tissue. Endocrinology 2007;148:1550–60.
55. Rossi J, Balthasar N, Olson D, et al. Melanocortin-4 receptors expressed by cholinergic neurons regulate energy balance and glucose homeostasis. Cell Metab 2011;13:195–204.
56. Butler AA, Marks DL, Fan W, et al. Melanocortin-4 receptor is required for acute homeostatic responses to increased dietary fat. Nat Neurosci 2001;4:605–11.
57. van deWall E, Leshan R, Xu AW, et al. Collective and individual functions of leptin receptor modulated neurons controlling metabolism and ingestion. Endocrinology 2008;149:1773–85.
58. Balthasar N, Coppari R, McMinn J, et al. Leptin receptor signaling in POMC neurons is required for normal body weight homeostasis. Neuron 2004;42: 983–91.

59. Davis TR, Mayer J. Imperfect homeothermia in the hereditary obese-hyperglycemic syndrome of mice. Am J Physiol 1954;177:222–6.

60. Trayhurn P, Thurlby PL, James WP. Thermogenic defect in pre-obese ob/ob mice. Nature 1977;266:60–2.

61. Trayhurn P, Thurlby PL, James WP. A defective response to cold in the obese (obob) mouse and the obese Zucker (fafa) rat [proceedings]. Proc Nutr Soc 1976;35:133A.

62. Joosten HF, van der Kroon PH. Role of the thyroid in the development of the obese-hyperglycemic syndrome in mice (ob ob). Metabolism 1974;23:425–36.

63. Commins SP, Watson PM, Padgett MA, et al. Induction of uncoupling protein expression in brown and white adipose tissue by leptin. Endocrinology 1999; 140:292–300.

64. Himms-Hagen J. Defective brown adipose tissue thermogenesis in obese mice. Int J Obes 1985;9(Suppl 2):17–24.

65. Rafael J, Herling AW. Leptin effect in ob/ob mice under thermoneutral conditions depends not necessarily on central satiation. Am J Physiol Regul Integr Comp Physiol 2000;278:R790–5.

66. Commins SP, Watson PM, Frampton IC, et al. Leptin selectively reduces white adipose tissue in mice via a UCP1-dependent mechanism in brown adipose tissue. Am J Physiol Endocrinol Metab 2001;280:E372–7.

67. Minokoshi Y, Alquier T, Furukawa N, et al. AMP-kinase regulates food intake by responding to hormonal and nutrient signals in the hypothalamus. Nature 2004; 428:569–74.

68. Pulinilkunnil T, He H, Kong D, et al. Adrenergic regulation of AMP-activated protein kinase in brown adipose tissue in vivo. J Biol Chem 2011;286: 8798–809.

69. Minokoshi Y, Kim YB, Peroni OD, et al. Leptin stimulates fatty-acid oxidation by activating AMP-activated protein kinase. Nature 2002;415:339–43.

70. Rosenbaum M, Goldsmith R, Bloomfield D, et al. Low-dose leptin reverses skeletal muscle, autonomic, and neuroendocrine adaptations to maintenance of reduced weight. J Clin Invest 2005;115:3579–86.

71. Zhang Y, Kerman IA, Laque A, et al. Leptin-receptor-expressing neurons in the dorsomedial hypothalamus and median preoptic area regulate sympathetic brown adipose tissue circuits. J Neurosci 2011;31:1873–84.

72. Enriori PJ, Sinnayah P, Simonds SE, et al. Leptin action in the dorsomedial hypothalamus increases sympathetic tone to brown adipose tissue in spite of systemic leptin resistance. J Neurosci 2011;31:12189–97.

73. Haynes WG, Morgan DA, Walsh SA, et al. Receptor-mediated regional sympathetic nerve activation by leptin. J Clin Invest 1997;100:270–8.

74. Mark AL, Agassandian K, Morgan DA, et al. Leptin signaling in the nucleus tractus solitarii increases sympathetic nerve activity to the kidney. Hypertension 2009;53:375–80.

75. Skibicka KP, Grill HJ. Hindbrain leptin stimulation induces anorexia and hyperthermia mediated by hindbrain melanocortin receptors. Endocrinology 2009; 150:1705–11.

76. Hermann GE, Barnes MJ, Rogers RC. Leptin and thyrotropin-releasing hormone: cooperative action in the hindbrain to activate brown adipose thermogenesis. Brain Res 2006;1117:118–24.

77. Rogers RC, McDougal DH, Hermann GE. Leptin amplifies the action of thyrotropin-releasing hormone in the solitary nucleus: an in vitro calcium imaging study. Brain Res 2011;1385:47–55.

78. Coppola A, Liu ZW, Andrews ZB, et al. A central thermogenic-like mechanism in feeding regulation: an interplay between arcuate nucleus T3 and UCP2. Cell Metab 2007;5:21–33.

79. Lopez M, Varela L, Vazquez MJ, et al. Hypothalamic AMPK and fatty acid metabolism mediate thyroid regulation of energy balance. Nat Med 2010;16: 1001–8.

80. Whittle AJ, Carobbio S, Martins L, et al. BMP8B increases brown adipose tissue thermogenesis through both central and peripheral actions. Cell 2012;149: 871–85.

81. Klaus S, Keipert S, Rossmeisl M, et al. Augmenting energy expenditure by mitochondrial uncoupling: a role of AMP-activated protein kinase. Genes Nutr 2012;7:369–86.

82. Bi S, Robinson BM, Moran TH. Acute food deprivation and chronic food restriction differentially affect hypothalamic NPY mRNA expression. Am J Physiol Regul Integr Comp Physiol 2003;285:R1030–6.

83. Li C, Chen P, Smith MS. The acute suckling stimulus induces expression of neuropeptide Y (NPY) in cells in the dorsomedial hypothalamus and increases NPY expression in the arcuate nucleus. Endocrinology 1998;139:1645–52.

84. Guan XM, Yu H, Trumbauer M, et al. Induction of neuropeptide Y expression in dorsomedial hypothalamus of diet-induced obese mice. Neuroreport 1998;9:3415–9.

85. Kesterson RA, Huszar D, Lynch CA, et al. Induction of neuropeptide Y gene expression in the dorsal medial hypothalamic nucleus in two models of the agouti obesity syndrome. Mol Endocrinol 1997;11:630–7.

86. Tritos NA, Elmquist JK, Mastaitis JW, et al. Characterization of expression of hypo-thalamic appetite-regulating peptides in obese hyperleptinemic brown adipose tissue-deficient (uncoupling protein-promoter-driven diphtheria toxin A) mice. Endocrinology 1998;139:4634–41.

87. Guan XM, Yu H, Van der Ploeg LH. Evidence of altered hypothalamic pro-opiomelanocortin/neuropeptide Y mRNA expression in tubby mice. Brain Res Mol Brain Res 1998;59:273–9.

88. Chao PT, Yang L, Aja S, et al. Knockdown of NPY expression in the dorsomedial hypothalamus promotes development of brown adipocytes and prevents diet-induced obesity. Cell Metab 2011;13:573–83.

89. Cinti S. The adipose organ at a glance. Dis Model Mech 2012;5:588–94.

90. Seale P, Bjork B, Yang W, et al. PRDM16 controls a brown fat/skeletal muscle switch. Nature 2008;454:961–7.

91. Richard D, Picard F. Brown fat biology and thermogenesis. Front Biosci 2011;16: 1233–60.

92. Petrovic N, Walden TB, Shabalina IG, et al. Chronic peroxisome proliferator-activated receptor gamma (PPARgamma) activation of epididymally derived white adipocyte cultures reveals a population of thermogenically competent, UCP1-containing adipocytes molecularly distinct from classic brown adipo-cytes. J Biol Chem 2010;285:7153–64.

93. Schulz TJ, Huang TL, Tran TT, et al. Identification of inducible brown adipocyte progenitors residing in skeletal muscle and white fat. Proc Natl Acad Sci U S A 2011;108:143–8.

94. Seale P, Conroe HM, Estall J, et al. Prdm16 determines the thermogenic program of subcutaneous white adipose tissue in mice. J Clin Invest 2011; 121:96–105.

95. Wu J, Bostrom P, Sparks LM, et al. Beige adipocytes are a distinct type of ther-mogenic fat cell in mouse and human. Cell 2012;150:366–76.

96. Stephens M, Ludgate M, Rees DA. Brown fat and obesity: the next big thing? Clin Endocrinol (Oxf) 2011;74:661–70.

97. Thomas C, Auwerx J, Schoonjans K. Bile acids and the membrane bile acid receptor TGR5–connecting nutrition and metabolism. Thyroid 2008;18:167–74.

98. Silvestri C, Ligresti A, Di M, et al. Peripheral effects of the endocannabinoid system in energy homeostasis: adipose tissue, liver and skeletal muscle. Rev Endocr Metab Disord 2011;12:153–62.

99. Vegiopoulos A, Muller-Decker K, Strzoda D, et al. Cyclooxygenase-2 controls energy homeostasis in mice by de novo recruitment of brown adipocytes. Science 2010;328:1158–61.

100. Madsen L, Pedersen LM, Lillefosse HH, et al. UCP1 induction during recruitment of brown adipocytes in white adipose tissue is dependent on cyclooxygenase activity. PLoS One 2010;5:e11391.

101. Ishibashi J, Seale P. Medicine. Beige can be slimming. Science 2010;328: 1113–4.

102. Dailey L, Ambrosetti D, Mansukhani A, et al. Mechanisms underlying differential responses to FGF signaling. Cytokine Growth Factor Rev 2005;16:233–47.

103. Mejhert N, Galitzky J, Pettersson AT, et al. Mapping of the fibroblast growth factors in human white adipose tissue. J Clin Endocrinol Metab 2010;95:2451–7.

104. Jonker JW, Suh JM, Atkins AR, et al. A PPARgamma-FGF1 axis is required for adaptive adipose remodelling and metabolic homeostasis. Nature 2012;485: 391–4.

105. Goetz R, Beenken A, Ibrahimi OA, et al. Molecular insights into the klotho-dependent, endocrine mode of action of fibroblast growth factor 19 subfamily members. Mol Cell Biol 2007;27:3417–28.

106. Dutchak PA, Katafuchi T, Bookout AL, et al. Fibroblast growth factor-21 regulates PPARgamma activity and the antidiabetic actions of thiazolidinediones. Cell 2012;148:556–67.

107. Canto C, Auwerx J. Cell biology. FGF21 takes a fat bite. Science 2012;336: 675–6.

108. Fisher FM, Kleiner S, Douris N, et al. FGF21 regulates PGC-1alpha and browning of white adipose tissues in adaptive thermogenesis. Genes Dev 2012;26: 271–81.

109. Wei W, Dutchak PA, Wang X, et al. Fibroblast growth factor 21 promotes bone loss by potentiating the effects of peroxisome proliferator-activated receptor gamma. Proc Natl Acad Sci U S A 2012;109:3143–8.

110. Chen G, Deng C, Li YP. TGF-beta and BMP signaling in osteoblast differentiation and bone formation. Int J Biol Sci 2012;8:272–88.

111. Ducy P, Zhang R, Geoffroy V, et al. Osf2/Cbfa1: a transcriptional activator of osteoblast differentiation. Cell 1997;89:747–54.

112. Tseng YH, Kokkotou E, Schulz TJ, et al. New role of bone morphogenetic protein 7 in brown adipogenesis and energy expenditure. Nature 2008;454:1000–4.

113. Sun Z. Cardiovascular responses to cold exposure. Front Biosci (Elite Ed) 2010; 2:495–503.

114. Sengenes C, Berlan M, De Glisezinski I, et al. Natriuretic peptides: a new lipolytic pathway in human adipocytes. FASEB J 2000;14:1345–51.

115. Haas B, Mayer P, Jennissen K, et al. Protein kinase G controls brown fat cell differentiation and mitochondrial biogenesis. Sci Signal 2009;2:ra78.

116. Bordicchia M, Liu D, Amri EZ, et al. Cardiac natriuretic peptides act via p38 MAPK to induce the brown fat thermogenic program in mouse and human adipocytes. J Clin Invest 2012;122:1022–36.

117. Bostrom P, Wu J, Jedrychowski MP, et al. A PGC1-alpha-dependent myokine that drives brown-fat-like development of white fat and thermogenesis. Nature 2012;481:463–8.
118. Nilsson SK, Heeren J, Olivecrona G, et al. Apolipoprotein A-V; a potent triglyceride reducer. Atherosclerosis 2011;219:15–21.
119. Davies BS, Beigneux AP, Fong LG, et al. New wrinkles in lipoprotein lipase biology. Curr Opin Lipidol 2012;23:35–42.
120. Heeren J, Niemeier A, Merkel M, et al. Endothelial-derived lipoprotein lipase is bound to postprandial triglyceride-rich lipoproteins and mediates their hepatic clearance in vivo. J Mol Med (Berl) 2002;80:576–84.
121. Bartelt A, Bruns OT, Reimer R, et al. Brown adipose tissue activity controls triglyceride clearance. Nat Med 2011;17:200–5.
122. Bartelt A, Merkel M, Heeren J. A new, powerful player in lipoprotein metabolism: brown adipose tissue. J Mol Med (Berl) 2012;90:887–93.
123. Williams KJ, Fisher EA. Globular warming: how fat gets to the furnace. Nat Med 2011;17:157–9.
124. Bartelt A, Heeren J. The holy grail of metabolic disease: brown adipose tissue. Curr Opin Lipidol 2012;23:190–5.
125. Zechner R, Zimmermann R, Eichmann TO, et al. FAT SIGNALS–lipases and lipolysis in lipid metabolism and signaling. Cell Metab 2012;15:279–91.
126. Haemmerle G, Moustafa T, Woelkart G, et al. ATGL-mediated fat catabolism regulates cardiac mitochondrial function via PPAR-alpha and PGC-1. Nat Med 2011;17:1076–85.
127. Lowell BB, Spiegelman BM. Towards a molecular understanding of adaptive thermogenesis. Nature 2000;404:652–60.
128. Hondares E, Rosell M, Diaz-Delfin J, et al. Peroxisome proliferator-activated receptor alpha (PPARalpha) induces PPARgamma coactivator 1alpha (PGC-1alpha) gene expression and contributes to thermogenic activation of brown fat: involvement of PRDM16. J Biol Chem 2011;286:43112–22.
129. Nedergaard J, Bengtsson T, Cannon B. New powers of brown fat: fighting the metabolic syndrome. Cell Metab 2011;13:238–40.
130. Enerback S, Jacobsson A, Simpson EM, et al. Mice lacking mitochondrial uncoupling protein are cold-sensitive but not obese. Nature 1997;387:90–4.
131. Ukropec J, Anunciado RP, Ravussin Y, et al. UCP1-independent thermogenesis in white adipose tissue of cold-acclimated Ucp1-/- mice. J Biol Chem 2006;281:31894–908.
132. Feldmann HM, Golozoubova V, Cannon B, et al. UCP1 ablation induces obesity and abolishes diet-induced thermogenesis in mice exempt from thermal stress by living at thermoneutrality. Cell Metab 2009;9:203–9.
133. Yamada T, Katagiri H, Ishigaki Y, et al. Signals from intra-abdominal fat modulate insulin and leptin sensitivity through different mechanisms: neuronal involvement in food-intake regulation. Cell Metab 2006;3:223–9.
134. Hany TF, Gharehpapagh E, Kamel EM, et al. Brown adipose tissue: a factor to consider in symmetrical tracer uptake in the neck and upper chest region. Eur J Nucl Med Mol Imaging 2002;29:1393–8.
135. van Marken Lichtenbelt WD. Brown adipose tissue and the regulation of non-shivering thermogenesis. Curr Opin Clin Nutr Metab Care 2012;15:547–52.
136. Nedergaard J, Bengtsson T, Cannon B. Three years with adult human brown adipose tissue. Ann N Y Acad Sci 2010;1212:E20–36.
137. Cypess AM, Lehman S, Williams G, et al. Identification and importance of brown adipose tissue in adult humans. N Engl J Med 2009;360:1509–17.

138. Virtanen KA, Lidell ME, Orava J, et al. Functional brown adipose tissue in healthy adults. N Engl J Med 2009;360:1518–25.

139. Enerback S. Human brown adipose tissue. Cell Metab 2010;11:248–52.

140. Chechi K, Blanchard PG, Mathieu P, et al. Brown fat like gene expression in the epicardial fat depot correlates with circulating HDL-cholesterol and triglycerides in patients with coronary artery disease. Int J Cardiol 2012. [Epub ahead of print].

141. Ouellet V, Labbe SM, Blondin DP, et al. Brown adipose tissue oxidative metabolism contributes to energy expenditure during acute cold exposure in humans. J Clin Invest 2012;122:545–52.

142. Orava J, Nuutila P, Lidell ME, et al. Different metabolic responses of human brown adipose tissue to activation by cold and insulin. Cell Metab 2011;14: 272–9.

143. Cypess AM, Chen YC, Sze C, et al. Cold but not sympathomimetics activates human brown adipose tissue in vivo. Proc Natl Acad Sci U S A 2012;109: 10001–5.

Brain Insulin and Leptin Signaling in Metabolic Control

From Animal Research to Clinical Application

Thomas Scherer, MD[a],*, Hendrik Lehnert, MD[b],
Manfred Hallschmid, PhD[c,d]

KEYWORDS

- Leptin • Insulin • Brain • Metabolism • Energy homeostasis
- Intranasal administration

KEY POINTS

- Brain insulin and leptin signaling are implicated in regulating key processes of metabolic function, such as food intake, appetite, energy expenditure, and nutrient partitioning.
- Both hormones act as negative feedback signals to the brain to maintain energy balance.
- Behavioral and functional neuroimaging studies support the notion that both peptide hormones affect human brain function, including memory formation and emotional state.
- Brain insulin signaling may be implicated in the pathophysiology of neurodegenerative diseases, such as Alzheimer disease.
- In the obese state, the brain's sensitivity for insulin and leptin is reduced, which hampers the efficacy of both signals to reduce food intake, lose weight, and improve glycemic control.
- In humans and rodents, peptide hormones, such as insulin and leptin, can easily be targeted to the brain along the olfactory system via the intranasal (IN) route of administration.
- Modulating brain insulin and leptin signaling may represent a future therapeutic option in the treatment of diabetes and obesity and also cognitive impairments.

INTRODUCTION

Paleontologic evidence indicates that changes in dietary composition benefited brain growth and the associated development of higher cognitive capacity during human evolution.[1,2] Moreover, hormones secreted from the digestive system are potent

Disclosure Statement: The authors have no conflict of interest.
[a] Division of Endocrinology and Metabolism, Department of Internal Medicine III, Medical University of Vienna, Waehringer Guertel 18-20, Vienna 1090, Austria; [b] Department of Internal Medicine I, University of Luebeck, Ratzeburger Allee 160, Luebeck 23538, Germany; [c] Department of Medical Psychology and Behavioral Neurobiology, University of Tuebingen, Otfried-Mueller-Strasse 25, Tuebingen 72076, Germany; [d] Institute for Diabetes Research and Metabolic Diseases of the Helmholtz Centre Munich, University of Tuebingen (Paul Langerhans Institute Tuebingen), Otfried-Mueller-Strasse 10, Tuebingen D-72076, Germany
* Corresponding author.
E-mail address: thomas.scherer@meduniwien.ac.at

modulators of central nervous functions, affecting not only ingestive behavior but also mood and memory formation.[1,3] The notion that, vice versa, the central nervous system (CNS) could be involved in the regulation of energy metabolism dates back as far as the nineteenth century. Claude Bernard reported that a "piqûre" at the base of the fourth ventricle in rabbits led to glucosuria and, in his words, "artificial diabetes."[4] In the 1940s, hypothalamic lesion studies in rodents suggested that the hypothalamus represents the key brain region where control of satiety and energy homeostasis are anatomically integrated.[5] In recent years, the concept of brain control of energy metabolism has progressed considerably and received a particular boost by the discovery of leptin.[6] Leptin is an adipocyte-derived hormone that crosses the blood-brain barrier (BBB) via a saturable transport.[7,8] It functions as an adiposity signal that communicates energy storage levels to the brain, which in turn regulates food intake and energy homeostasis.[9] Leptin administration in leptin-deficient humans and rodents reduces food intake and adiposity.[10,11] In addition, brain leptin signaling has functions that go beyond its ability to alter food intake. It is implicated in the regulation of glucose homeostasis,[12] lipid metabolism,[13] reward-related behavior,[14] and the processing of the reward value of nutrients.[15] Leptin also positively controls reproductive function,[16,17] acting as a pivotal hormonal energy signal that links nutritional status and reproduction.[18] Furthermore, the hormone modulates synaptic plasticity in the hippocampus[19] and has been shown to improve depression-like behavior in animals,[20] suggesting that impaired central nervous leptin signaling might contribute to the association between obesity and depression.[21]

Similar to leptin, insulin, despite being secreted by pancreatic β cells, also circulates approximately in proportion to body fat,[22] particularly in the prediabetic state, and is considered an adiposity signal that suppresses food intake. This was first demonstrated by intracerebroventricular (ICV) application of insulin in baboons more than 3 decades ago.[23] Although there is some evidence for local insulin production in the CNS,[24] it is generally believed that peripheral insulin, like leptin, enters the brain by crossing the BBB via a saturable transport system.[25,26] Brain insulin signaling has also been implicated in the regulation of glucose and lipid homeostasis[27,28] and the nonhomeostatic control of food intake by reward processing[14,29,30] as well as in learning,[31] synaptic plasticity,[32] and a variety of other functions, such as reproductive control[33] and growth,[34] and might likewise play a pathophysiologic role in neurodegenerative diseases.[35]

The above-mentioned studies that shaped the concept of leptin and insulin brain signaling were mainly performed in rodents. Neuronal insulin and leptin signaling can be manipulated locally by stereotaxic infusion of the respective hormone via a pre-implanted cannula, which targets either the ventricular system or the mediobasal hypothalamus (MBH). Both neuronal insulin and leptin receptor signaling are able to affect peripheral hormone concentrations by, for example, modulating insulin secretion from the pancreas.[36,37] Thus, in order to isolate the brain effects of insulin and leptin, it is key to control for circulating glucose and insulin levels by using euglycemic pancreatic clamp studies. Targeted peptide delivery to the human CNS without changing peripheral insulin and glucose concentrations is particularly difficult, because a direct route of delivery seems to be missing. Although it is possible to use an intravenous approach for peptides that are selectively transported across the BBB to induce CNS effects,[38] these peptides inevitably activate their peripheral receptors, if present. In the case of insulin, this leads to hypoglycemia, which itself triggers a strong sympathetic nervous system (SNS) response. Even if this is prevented by a continuous glucose infusion, the systemic application of insulin does not allow differentiation between peripherally and centrally mediated effects of the infused hormone.

In humans, these experimental limitations can be overcome via the IN route of administration (reviewed by Ott and colleagues[39]), which achieves effective delivery of insulin and other peptides to the CNS, presumably via the olfactory system,[40] without relevant uptake into systemic circulation.[41] Currently, studies on IN leptin administration in humans are lacking. It is likely, however, that IN delivery of leptin also is a feasible approach in humans because rodent studies show that IN leptin administration reduces food intake in rats without causing relevant changes in circulating leptin levels.[42–44] This article reviews the current evidence for metabolic effects of brain insulin and leptin signaling in humans and animals, with a particular emphasis on human studies.

CONTROL OF METABOLISM BY CENTRAL NERVOUS INSULIN SIGNALING

Insulin has well-characterized systemic effects: it decreases postprandial blood glucose concentrations by reducing hepatic gluconeogenesis as well as increasing glycogen synthesis and glucose uptake into muscle and white adipose tissue (WAT). Furthermore, insulin is the major antilipolytic hormone.[45] It stimulates de novo lipogenesis in WAT and the liver and reduces hepatic triglyceride secretion, thus promoting lipid retention and storage.[46,47] These classic functions of insulin used to be primarily attributed to the direct effects of insulin, which are mediated via the insulin receptor expressed on the respective organ of action. Several recent rodent studies suggest, however, that insulin also indirectly conveys some of these metabolic functions by binding to its neuronal receptors, thereby modulating autonomic nervous system outflow to peripheral organs. These effects are complementary to the peripheral effects of insulin and may be interpreted as functional redundancy in physiology. For example, short-term brain insulin infusion studies combined with basal euglycemic pancreatic clamps have demonstrated that brain insulin signaling suppresses hepatic glucose production[27,48] independent of circulating insulin and glucose levels. Insulin seems to elicit these effects by opening ATP-dependent potassium (K_{ATP}) channels in the MBH.[49] Conversely, the lack of brain insulin receptors in a genetic knockout model leads to a mild diabetic phenotype when these mice age.[33] In addition, restoration of hepatic insulin signaling in the presence of a hypothalamic insulin-signaling defect is insufficient to restore glucose homeostasis.[50] Furthermore, hypothalamic insulin action suppresses WAT lipolytic flux and increases de novo lipogenesis in rats via a dampening of the SNS outflow to WAT, whereas pharmacologic blockade or brain insulin receptor deficiency unrestrains lipolysis.[28]

Insulin Signaling in Larger Mammals

So far, however, it is unclear whether these brain regulatory pathways are also relevant in larger mammals, such as humans. The role of CNS insulin signaling in mediating the acute effects of insulin to suppress hepatic glucose production has recently been challenged. Although short-term infusion studies in dogs supported the notion that the canine brain is also able to sense a rise in systemic insulin, brain insulin action only mildly reduced net hepatic glucose output, which was largely due to changes in hepatic glucose uptake and glycogen storage.[51] Despite a reduction in hepatic gluconeogenic gene expression, hepatic glucose production was unchanged when insulin was given ICV in dogs.[51] However, these studies are only in a position to evaluate the acute effects of brain insulin on hepatic glucose metabolism. The impact of a chronic lack of brain insulin signaling on glucose homeostasis as implicated by several genetic mouse models[33,50,52] cannot be deducted from these experiments. Furthermore, differences in the experimental design, especially regarding the clamp design and the sampling period, might also have contributed to the discrepancies between rodent and canine studies (reviewed by Ramnanan and colleagues[53]).

Evidence for Brain Insulin Action in Humans

In humans, a recent study showed that the orally administered K_{ATP} channel opener, diazoxide, reduces hepatic glucose production as assessed by tracer dilution techniques during a basal insulin clamp in healthy nondiabetic human subjects.[54] An analogous experiment in rats under similar conditions replicated this effect. Furthermore, ICV infusion of the K_{ATP} channel blocker, glibenclamide, abolished the ability of oral diazoxide to reduce hepatic glucose output in rats, strongly suggesting that the effects of the K_{ATP} channel activator are centrally mediated. This study does not prove the presence of a brain-liver axis in humans because systemic effects after oral administration of diazoxide cannot be entirely ruled out: before the clamp was started, insulin levels were slightly decreased by diazoxide, which peripherally acts as potent inhibitor of insulin secretion. This is the first experimental attempt, however, to assess whether the brain can independently regulate hepatic glucose metabolism in humans using the pancreatic clamp technique combined with stable isotope tracers. It is tempting to speculate that an IN route of delivery would have allowed a further dose reduction and a more targeted delivery of diazoxide to the brain without changes in baseline insulin levels. To the authors' knowledge, such a study has not been performed, although several other experiments in humans were conducted that relied on the IN delivery of insulin. Unfortunately, none of these studies used tracer dilution techniques to assess glucose flux directly.

A recent study showed that a boost in brain insulin signaling might improve peripheral insulin sensitivity.[55] Two hours after an IN insulin bolus, the homeostasis model assessment (HOMA) score, which is calculated using blood glucose and serum insulin levels and indicates the degree of insulin resistance, was significantly lower compared with that of the placebo group. Circulating glucose levels were likewise decreased, which is consistent with other reports,[56,57] suggesting that IN insulin reduces circulating blood glucose possibly via central nervous action. This study has some limitations, however: a high IN insulin dose was chosen, which may have partially leaked into circulation and caused an early peak in systemic insulin, whereas lower IN insulin doses have been shown not to induce relevant alterations in circulating insulin.[58,139] Although the changes in glucose metabolism persisted after insulin levels had returned to normal values, systemic effects of insulin cannot be entirely excluded. Furthermore, the HOMA score is validated for fasting conditions and not when insulin levels are acutely altered. Nevertheless, the changes in the HOMA score were correlated with brain activity in several brain regions, including the hypothalamus, putamen, orbitofrontal cortex, and right insula, as assessed by functional MRI (fMRI), indicating that part of the effects of IN insulin on peripheral metabolism might have been mediated by the brain.

Brain Insulin and WAT Metabolism

With regard to the control of WAT lipolysis by central nervous insulin reported in rats,[28] a recent human study has yielded preliminary evidence that IN insulin might be able to reduce free fatty acid levels independent of peripheral insulin signaling.[57] Although, again, peripheral insulin levels spiked shortly after IN insulin application, correlational analyses imply that the decrease in free fatty acid levels was unrelated to the changes in circulating insulin. Similar to the animal studies (described previously) where brain insulin suppressed lipolysis by reducing SNS outflow to WAT,[28] IN insulin in humans is able to reduce SNS activity as assessed by circulating epinephrine.[56] This suggests that brain insulin signaling in humans is directly linked to autonomic nervous system activity, although in another study muscular sympathetic nervous activity was not affected by IN insulin.[59] Taken together, further studies using tracer dilution techniques are required to fully assess whether brain insulin signaling regulates whole-body glucose and lipid metabolism in humans.

Brain Insulin Action and Energy Balance

Rodent studies have indicated that brain insulin signaling is implicated in not only the regulation of food intake[60–62] but also energy expenditure.[63] In contrast to its effect on WAT, CNS insulin signaling stimulates SNS outflow to the brown adipose tissue compartment.[64] The same seems to hold true for humans, where IN insulin administration has been shown to increase postprandial energy expenditure in healthy male individuals.[57] There is a growing body of literature regarding brain insulin control of food intake in humans: an IN insulin bolus acutely reduced energy intake in male subjects, whereas female subjects remained unaffected,[65] and similar sex differences were also observed in rats.[60] Likewise, chronic application of IN insulin over 2 months caused a reduction in body fat and weight circumference in healthy male but not female subjects.[66] Cognitive components of satiety seem to be affected as well inasmuch as IN insulin reduces neuronal activity in several brain regions when food-related visual stimuli are processed.[67] This was observed in male and female subjects alike. Furthermore, postprandial administration of IN insulin intensified meal-related satiety and reduced subsequent intake of highly palatable snacks in women.[68] In summary, these data indicate that brain insulin signaling likely plays a role in modulating food intake, satiety, and adiposity in humans.

Cognitive Effects of Brain Insulin

Besides homeostatic and nonhomeostatic mechanisms, memory for food intake critically contributes to the control of ingestive behavior in humans.[69] This is highlighted by the observation that amnesic patients with hippocampal lesions eat multiple meals if left unaware of preceding food intake.[70,71] Against this background, the role of brain insulin extends to the cognitive domain, including the formation of hippocampus-dependent memory. The hippocampus is highly relevant for the formation and maintenance of declarative memory (ie, memory for facts and episodes that is accessible to conscious recollection).[72] Several studies indicate that insulin modulates changes in hippocampal synaptic plasticity by potentiating long-term depression and potentiation, respectively, at different synapses.[73] In addition, insulin may promote glucose utilization of neuronal networks.[74] Although in general, glucose transport to the CNS is assumed insulin independent,[75,76] prolonged hyperinsulinemia in rodents affects glucose metabolism in regions like the anterior hypothalamus and the basolateral amygdala.[77] In line with these findings, central nervous administration of the hormone via the IN route has been found, in studies in healthy humans, to improve memory functions.[31,65,78] Beneficial effects of IN insulin on declarative memory have likewise been demonstrated in subjects suffering from amnestic symptoms (eg, due to Alzheimer disease).[79–81] Furthermore, CNS insulin signaling also seems to contribute to emotional functions: Lentivirus-mediated downregulation of hypothalamic insulin receptor expression in rats elicits depressive and anxiety-like behaviors,[82] whereas improvements in self-rated mood were observed in healthy humans after 8 weeks of IN insulin administration.[31]

Brain Insulin Resistance in Humans

In obese and insulin-resistant humans, brain insulin signaling is impaired. Although systemic hyperinsulinemia elicits changes in cortical activity, as assessed by magnetoencephalography in healthy lean women and men, this effect is reduced in obese subjects and negatively correlated with fat mass.[83] Also, 8 weeks of IN insulin administration remained without effect on fat mass in obese subjects.[84] These findings might be interpreted in terms of cerebral insulin resistance, which could be due to a defect in the transporter that carries insulin across the BBB, a defect on the level of the insulin receptor or its downstream signaling cascade. Short-term overfeeding in rodents also leads to impaired brain insulin action both with respect to hepatic glucose control[85,86] and WAT lipolysis.[87] Because brain insulin action is lost even when insulin is directly delivered to its target regions by stereotaxic infusions in rats,[86,87] a transporter defect is likely not the predominant mechanism. Similarly, short-term caloric excess in human studies induces isolated hepatic insulin resistance[88,89] that, according to the rodent studies (cited previously)[27,49] might be mediated by impaired brain insulin action. High-calorie intake and obesity have been associated with brain insulin signaling defects on the level of the receptor,[86] increased endoplasmatic reticulum stress in the MBH, and hypothalamic inflammation and gliosis.[90,91] Hypothalamic gliosis is also present in obese human subjects, as recently shown by brain MRI.[90] Epidemiologic findings indicate an association between obesity and diabetes and cognitive impairments, including dementia.[92] Furthermore, poor glycemic control in type 2 diabetic patients, as assessed by glycated hemoglobin, inversely correlates with hippocampal volume.[93] It is currently being discussed whether dysfunctional brain insulin signaling might be a common mechanism of metabolic and cognitive disorders.[94] Because brain insulin sensitivity in humans is positively associated with loss of body weight and adiposity due to lifestyle intervention,[95] enhancing brain insulin signaling or compensating for the signaling defect might offer a feasible approach to improve whole-body metabolic control. The IN route for drug delivery might aid by administering compounds in a more targeted fashion. In addition, IN insulin seems to have an exceptional safety profile, because the studies published so far have reported almost no risk for developing systemic hypoglycemia, a common problem of several antidiabetic drug treatments.

CONTROL OF METABOLISM BY CENTRAL NERVOUS LEPTIN SIGNALING

Although insulin and leptin are both considered anorexic signals communicating whole-body energy levels to the brain to orchestrate food intake and energy expenditure,[9] some brain effects of these hormones are different (extensively reviewed by Scherer and Buettner[96]). Compared with insulin, brain leptin signaling has opposing acute effects on glucose and lipid metabolism. It promotes gluconeogenesis[97] and stimulates lipolysis but blocks de novo lipogenesis in WAT.[13] Thus, according to the aforementioned studies, brain leptin signaling promotes catabolic processes opposing the fat-preserving properties of brain insulin. In the long run, these effects contribute to the ability of leptin to reduce adiposity. Although peripheral leptin receptors exist, the metabolic effects of leptin seem predominantly mediated via the brain, because (1) targeted reconstitution of the leptin receptor in the brain completely resolves the obese, hyperphagic, and diabetic phenotype of leptin receptor deficient db/db mice,[98] and (2) an inducible leptin receptor knockout in the periphery but not in the brain causes no obvious metabolic phenotype in mice.[99] In leptin-deficient humans with a missense mutation in the ob gene, leptin replacement reduced body mass index and increased satiety as well as neuronal activation in the prefrontal cortex[100] that plays a key role in behavioral control and dieting.[101] Marked differences after leptin treatment were also observed in striatal regions that are involved in regulating reward-related behavior.[102] Conversely, pausing the leptin therapy increased body mass index and enhanced brain activation in the gustatory cortex, a brain region that is highly activated in states of hunger.[103] Although patients with mutations in the *ob* gene are rare and obesity is classically associated with hyperleptinemia rather than leptin deficiency, these studies provide proof of principle that the leptin signal arising in the periphery is sensed and integrated not only in the rodent but also in the human brain.

Circulating Leptin Modulates Energy Balance

Besides its role as an adiposity signal that exerts anorexigenic effects in the regulation of food intake, leptin promotes energy expenditure. When the energy supply exceeds the current demands, leptin levels increase, blocking food intake and increasing energy expenditure, leading to a negative energy balance and restoring energy homeostasis. Conversely, *ob/ob* mice that lack the leptin gene are morbidly obese not only because of massive hyperphagia but also due to a reduction in metabolic rate, physical activity, and body temperature, all of which is reversible after leptin replacement.[10] Leptin treatment also leads to increased oxygen consumption and thermogenesis in nonmutant rodents.[104] It is, therefore, conceivable that a reduction in circulating leptin levels leads to energy preservation due to lower energy expenditure. In mice, starvation induces a marked decrease in leptin concentrations[105] and similar changes are observed in humans losing weight[106]: because leptin circulates in levels proportional to adiposity, weight loss results in lower plasma leptin concentrations and, hence, reduced energy expenditure.[107] Leptin levels that are persistently lower compared with baseline after losing weight and that do not revert to the initial concentrations for over a year[108] hamper interventions aiming at sustained weight loss by dietary regimens.[109] Apparently, the body perceives the relative hypoleptinemia as a state of starvation and energy deficiency and tries to preserve the original body weight. Leptin substitution after weight loss, in other words, compensation for the relative leptin deficiency, reverses these changes, enabling subjects to maintain their lower body weight.[107] These effects of exogenously administered leptin again are at least partially mediated via the brain: in a study by Rosenbaum and colleagues,[110] brain activity after presenting visual food cues was assessed by fMRI in humans before and after sustained weight loss with or without exogenous leptin treatment. Leptin treatment and weight loss both caused distinct changes in multiple brain regions involved in regulating food intake and satiety, such as the insula region, hypothalamus, amygdala, and brainstem. Strikingly, leptin treatment to improve weight maintenance after weight loss restored brain activity patterns to those assessed before losing weight, thus reinstating the initial, preweight loss, brain leptin signaling. Leptin substitution, which helps maintain a lower body weight, in conjunction with the finding that leptin reverses neuronal activity to preweight loss patterns, strongly suggest that brain leptin signaling plays a pivotal role in modulating satiety and cognitive control of food intake in the human brain.

Brain Leptin Regulation of Glucose Metabolism

Furthermore, it is conceivable that the anorexigenic and energy expenditure–promoting effects of leptin, in the long run, lead to reduced adiposity and eventually improved glucose control. In addition, chronic hyperleptinemia per se has clear glucose-lowering effects in normal rats.[111] Acute systemic leptin administration also regulates hepatic glucose metabolism independent of any changes in body weight. Systemic leptin injections in rats subjected to hyperinsulinemic clamp studies enhanced the effects of insulin and further reduced hepatic glucose production. Although the contribution of gluconeogenesis to hepatic glucose production increased, glycogenolysis was markedly reduced. Peripheral glucose fluxes were not altered.[112] These effects were almost completely replicated when leptin was administered ICV into the third ventricle at much lower doses in lean male rats, suggesting that brain leptin action is largely responsible for these effects.[12] Brain leptin has also been shown to influence glucose homeostasis in type 1 diabetes, a state of insulin deficiency. It was demonstrated in partially insulin-deficient rats that leptin can restore euglycemia,[113] and leptin overexpression completely rescued fatally ill mice suffering from autoimmune or chemically induced type 1 diabetes with severe, prolonged insulin deficiency,[114] an effect that was possibly due to leptin's ability to lower glucagon secretion.[115] Again, these effects were largely replicated when leptin was administered centrally and unrelated to changes in food intake.[116–118] A predominant CNS mechanism is further supported by leptin treatment as effective in insulin-deficient hepatocyte-specific leptin receptor knockout mice.[119] Taken together, these data suggest that leptin and, more specifically, brain leptin could be a potential antidiabetic therapeutic. However, 14 days of twice-daily subcutaneous leptin treatment did not enhance insulin sensitivity in obese patients with newly diagnosed type 2 diabetes, although the high treatment dose yielded a 150-fold increase in basal plasma concentrations.[120] Furthermore, obese, diabetic subjects who received a lower dose of subcutaneous leptin for 16 weeks showed only a moderate improvement in glycemic control.[121] Although these results might imply that leptin's effect on insulin sensitivity is more permissive than pivotal,[122] leptin's efficiency in these studies might have been hampered by the peripheral route of administration (discussed later). With regard to type 1 diabetes, there are no published study yet available; however, there is an ongoing clinical pilot trial that examines the effects of metreleptin in type 1 diabetic patients (NCT01268644, clinicaltrials.gov).

Brain Leptin and Hepatic Steatosis

The obese state is associated with many metabolic alterations, summarized under the term, metabolic syndrome. Besides central obesity, the metabolic syndrome is characterized by insulin resistance, dyslipidemia, high blood pressure, and low-grade inflammation. Furthermore, it is now known that hepatic steatosis, one of the most common liver pathologies, is closely associated with adiposity.[123] In rats, disrupted brain leptin signaling independently promotes hepatic lipid accumulation and hepatic steatosis, irrespective of changes in food intake or body weight.[124] Conversely, in the ob/ob mouse, systemic low-dose leptin treatment markedly increases triglyceride secretion rates, thereby reducing hepatic triglyceride content.[125] These effects of leptin again seem centrally mediated: although db/db mice and neuronal leptin receptor knockout mice have enlarged steatotic livers compared with controls, liver-specific leptin receptor knock-out mice show unaltered liver triglyceride content.[126] Similarly, humans with lipodystrophy, a rare condition where WAT is practically absent, also suffer from hypertriglyceridemia and massive hepatic steatosis due to ectopic lipid deposition. Because these patients have no WAT, leptin expression and circulating concentrations are low. In keeping with the notion that leptin deficiency promotes hepatic steatosis, restoration of normal leptin levels in these lipodystrophic patients considerably ameliorates their steatotic and dyslipidemic phenotype[127,128] despite that WAT is completely absent. So far, this represents the only Food and Drug Administration–authorized clinical application for the use of the recombinant human leptin, metreleptin, which is currently under an investigational new drug protocol.

CNS Leptin Resistance

In obese and diabetic subjects as well as in rodent models of diet-induced obesity, circulating leptin levels are usually increased, and further pharmacologic escalation of leptin concentrations has almost no effect on food intake, adiposity, or glucose homeostasis.[121,129] These findings indicate that in the obese and/or diabetic state, the organism develops leptin tolerance or resistance. This phenomenon is reminiscent of the aggravating insulin resistance of type 2 diabetic patients, which leads to a continuously increased insulin secretion due to higher demands and, eventually, to the necessity of exogenous insulin supplementation. Although brain insulin completely loses its ability to suppress hepatic glucose production and WAT lipolysis in overfed rats,[86,87] exogenous leptin restores hepatic glucose control in rats overfed for 3 days when administered ICV.[130] Thus, with regard to central control of glucose homeostasis, for brain leptin, in comparison with insulin, sensitivity at the receptor level seems preserved to some extent. Even after prolonged exposure to a high-fat diet, ICV leptin injections in mice can activate hypothalamic leptin signaling, although to a lesser extent than in regular chow controls, whereas intraperitoneal leptin injections are without effect.[131] It is assumed that blood-borne leptin does not reach the brain leptin receptor to elicit a signal, suggesting that a transporter defect at the BBB contributes to leptin resistance. This notion is supported by iodine-labeled leptin tracer studies in obese rats and mice, where leptin transport across the BBB is hampered compared with lean animals.[132,133] Although leptin distribution experiments have already been conducted in rats and primates using positron emission tomography, the sensitivity was not sufficient to detect tracer binding to hypothalamic leptin receptors.[134] Therefore, potential differences in the bioavailability of brain leptin cannot be verified yet in obese versus lean humans. It has already been demonstrated, however, that obese subjects have a decreased cerebrospinal fluid/serum leptin ratio compared with lean controls,[8] which supports the idea that in obese subjects leptin is not transported across the BBB in sufficient amounts, causing a relative deficiency in brain leptin signaling. Accordingly, peripheral leptin administration generally fails to improve metabolic control in obese subjects.[120,121,129]

In a rodent model of diet-induced obesity, 4 weeks of IN leptin administration reduced appetite and induced body weight loss to an extent that was comparable to the effects in lean rats.[42] The weight loss–promoting effects of IN leptin were supported by gene expression changes of hypothalamic neuropeptides classically related to appetite regulation. Although gene expression of the orexigenic neuropeptides, agouti-related peptide and neuropeptide Y, were suppressed by IN leptin treatment in both lean diet and high-fat diet–fed rats, pro-opiomelanocortin and cocaine- and amphetamine-regulated transcript, which both function as anorexigenic signals, were upregulated. Furthermore, IN-administered radiolabeled leptin preferentially reaches the hypothalamus, most likely via a direct transport of leptin from nose to brain because systemic hyperleptinemia does not block leptin uptake to the brain.[135] These promising findings suggest that direct targeting of leptin to the brain, circumventing a potential leptin transporter defect, might have therapeutic potential in the treatment of obesity. It remains to be determined, however, whether it is possible to overcome the leptin resistance of obese and diabetic subjects by directly administering leptin via the IN route.

LIMITATIONS AND CAVEATS

Despite the encouraging results of IN leptin administration in animal experiments, some limitations and caveats of the IN method of drug administration should be addressed. In light of the hyperleptinemia and hyperinsulinemia that accompany obesity and peripheral insulin resistance in type 2 diabetes, it might be argued that the reduction of cerebrospinal fluid leptin and insulin concentrations observed in obese subjects[8,136] could represent a protective mechanism that limits central nervous hyperinsulinemia and hyperleptinemia, preventing potentially detrimental consequences within the CNS. With regard to insulin, this assumption is in line with findings in healthy subjects where the induction of acute moderate euglycemic hyperinsulinemia triggered CNS inflammation and β-amyloid formation,[137] both of which are well-known risk factors for the development of cognitive impairments. The notion that brain hyperinsulinemia might promote central nervous insulin resistance is further supported by a recent in vitro study showing that prolonged (4–24 h) exposure of hypothalamic cells to high concentrations of insulin led to inactivation and degradation of the insulin receptor and insulin receptor substrate-1.[138]

Although the animal data (summarized previously) bode well for future translations to the clinical setting, the assumption that central nervous leptin and insulin play a crucial role in the regulation of, for example, adipocyte metabolism and whole-body glucose homeostasis in the human organism, still lacks experimental evidence. As yet, human studies that examined the effects of IN peptides mainly focused on behavioral parameters and central nervous readouts using a variety of methods, such as fMRI, positron emission tomography, and magnetic resonance spectroscopy of the brain, as well as electroncephalography and magnetoencephalography. Although several studies looked at peripheral readouts, such as blood glucose or lipid measurements, more reliable methods to assess glucose or lipid flux using stable isotope tracers were not used. Another complicating factor is that in some cases, especially when IN insulin was administered at high doses, insulin may have leaked into peripheral circulation, making it tricky to differentiate between central and peripheral effects. Against this background and considering that long-term clinical data on therapeutic and side effects of IN insulin and leptin in humans are not yet available, much work still needs to be done to fully evaluate the potential of IN peptide administration to the brain in the treatment of metabolic and cognitive disorders (**Fig. 1** provides an overview of IN insulin and leptin effects). Nevertheless, understanding

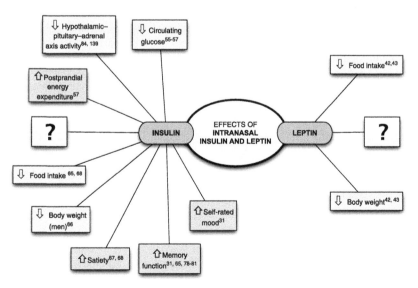

Fig. 1. Overview of metabolic and nonmetabolic effects of IN insulin and leptin in human and animal studies.

the physiology as well as pathophysiologic alterations of the CNS regulation of metabolism and nutrient partitioning in humans is of key relevance, and studies relying on the IN administration of insulin and leptin can be expected to prove valuable tools in this undertaking.

REFERENCES

1. Gomez-Pinilla F. Brain foods: the effects of nutrients on brain function. Nat Rev Neurosci 2008;9(7):568–78.
2. Crawford MA, Bloom M, Broadhurst CL, et al. Evidence for the unique function of docosahexaenoic acid during the evolution of the modern hominid brain. Lipids 1999;34(Suppl):S39–47.
3. McNay EC. Insulin and ghrelin: peripheral hormones modulating memory and hippocampal function. Curr Opin Pharmacol 2007;7(6):628–32.
4. Bernard C. Leçons de physiologie expérimentale appliquée à la médecine, faites au Collège de France, par m. Claude Bernard, vol. 1. Paris: Paris, J.B. Baillière et fils; 1855. p. 1855–56.
5. Hetherington AW, Ranson SW. Hypothalamic lesions and adiposity in the rat. Anat Rec 1940;78(2):149–72.
6. Halaas JL, Gajiwala KS, Maffei M, et al. Weight-reducing effects of the plasma protein encoded by the obese gene. Science 1995;269(5223):543–6.
7. Schwartz MW, Peskind E, Raskind M, et al. Cerebrospinal fluid leptin levels: relationship to plasma levels and to adiposity in humans. Nat Med 1996;2(5): 589–93.
8. Caro JF, Kolaczynski JW, Nyce MR, et al. Decreased cerebrospinal-fluid/serum leptin ratio in obesity: a possible mechanism for leptin resistance. Lancet 1996; 348(9021):159–61.
9. Schwartz MW, Woods SC, Porte D Jr, et al. Central nervous system control of food intake. Nature 2000;404(6778):661–71.
10. Pelleymounter MA, Cullen MJ, Baker MB, et al. Effects of the obese gene product on body weight regulation in ob/ob mice. Science 1995;269(5223):540–3.
11. Farooqi IS, Matarese G, Lord GM, et al. Beneficial effects of leptin on obesity, T cell hyporesponsiveness, and neuroendocrine/metabolic dysfunction of human congenital leptin deficiency. J Clin Invest 2002;110(8):1093–103.
12. Liu L, Karkanias GB, Morales JC, et al. Intracerebroventricular leptin regulates hepatic but not peripheral glucose fluxes. J Biol Chem 1998;273(47):31160–7.
13. Buettner C, Muse ED, Cheng A, et al. Leptin controls adipose tissue lipogenesis via central, STAT3-independent mechanisms. Nat Med 2008;14(6):667–75.
14. Davis JF, Choi DL, Benoit SC. Insulin, leptin and reward. Trends Endocrinol Metab 2010;21(2):68–74.
15. Domingos AI, Vaynshteyn J, Voss HU, et al. Leptin regulates the reward value of nutrient. Nat Neurosci 2011;14(12):1562–8.
16. Watanobe H, Suda T, Wikberg JE, et al. Evidence that physiological levels of circulating leptin exert a stimulatory effect on luteinizing hormone and prolactin surges in rats. Biochem Biophys Res Commun 1999;263(1):162–5.
17. Buettner C, Pocai A, Muse ED, et al. Critical role of STAT3 in leptin's metabolic actions. Cell Metab 2006;4(1):49–60.
18. Mantzoros CS. Role of leptin in reproduction. Ann N Y Acad Sci 2000;900: 174–83.
19. Shanley LJ, Irving AJ, Harvey J. Leptin enhances NMDA receptor function and modulates hippocampal synaptic plasticity. J Neurosci 2001;21(24):RC186.

20. Lu XY, Kim CS, Frazer A, et al. Leptin: a potential novel antidepressant. Proc Natl Acad Sci U S A 2006;103(5):1593–8.

21. Yamada N, Katsuura G, Ochi Y, et al. Impaired CNS leptin action is implicated in depression associated with obesity. Endocrinology 2011;152(7):2634–43.

22. Bagdade JD, Bierman EL, Porte D Jr. The significance of basal insulin levels in the evaluation of the insulin response to glucose in diabetic and nondiabetic subjects. J Clin Invest 1967;46(10):1549–57.

23. Porte D Jr, Woods SC. Regulation of food intake and body weight in insulin. Diabetologia 1981;20(Suppl):274–80.

24. Devaskar SU, Giddings SJ, Rajakumar PA, et al. Insulin gene expression and insulin synthesis in mammalian neuronal cells. J Biol Chem 1994;269(11): 8445–54.

25. Schwartz MW, Bergman RN, Kahn SE, et al. Evidence for entry of plasma insulin into cerebrospinal fluid through an intermediate compartment in dogs. Quantitative aspects and implications for transport. J Clin Invest 1991;88(4):1272–81.

26. Banks WA, Jaspan JB, Kastin AJ. Selective, physiological transport of insulin across the blood-brain barrier: novel demonstration by species-specific radioimmunoassays. Peptides 1997;18(8):1257–62.

27. Obici S, Zhang BB, Karkanias G, et al. Hypothalamic insulin signaling is required for inhibition of glucose production. Nat Med 2002;8(12):1376–82.

28. Scherer T, O'Hare J, Diggs-Andrews K, et al. Brain insulin controls adipose tissue lipolysis and lipogenesis. Cell Metab 2011;13(2):183–94.

29. Figlewicz DP, Bennett J, Evans SB, et al. Intraventricular insulin and leptin reverse place preference conditioned with high-fat diet in rats. Behav Neurosci 2004;118(3):479–87.

30. Figlewicz DP, Bennett JL, Naleid AM, et al. Intraventricular insulin and leptin decrease sucrose self-administration in rats. Physiol Behav 2006;89(4):611–6.

31. Benedict C, Hallschmid M, Hatke A, et al. Intranasal insulin improves memory in humans. Psychoneuroendocrinology 2004;29(10):1326–34.

32. Chiu SL, Chen CM, Cline HT. Insulin receptor signaling regulates synapse number, dendritic plasticity, and circuit function in vivo. Neuron 2008;58(5):708–19.

33. Bruning JC, Gautam D, Burks DJ, et al. Role of brain insulin receptor in control of body weight and reproduction. Science 2000;289(5487):2122–5.

34. Rulifson EJ, Kim SK, Nusse R. Ablation of insulin-producing neurons in flies: growth and diabetic phenotypes. Science 2002;296(5570):1118–20.

35. Schubert M, Gautam D, Surjo D, et al. Role for neuronal insulin resistance in neurodegenerative diseases. Proc Natl Acad Sci U S A 2004;101(9):3100–5.

36. Muzumdar R, Ma X, Yang X, et al. Physiologic effect of leptin on insulin secretion is mediated mainly through central mechanisms. FASEB J 2003;17(9):1130–2.

37. Chen M, Woods SC, Porte D Jr. Effect of cerebral intraventricular insulin on pancreatic insulin secretion in the dog. Diabetes 1975;24(10):910–4.

38. Wallum BJ, Taborsky GJ Jr, Porte D Jr, et al. Cerebrospinal fluid insulin levels increase during intravenous insulin infusions in man. J Clin Endocrinol Metab 1987;64(1):190–4.

39. Ott V, Benedict C, Schultes B, et al. Intranasal administration of insulin to the brain impacts cognitive function and peripheral metabolism. Diabetes Obes Metab 2012;14(3):214–21.

40. Thorne RG, Emory CR, Ala TA, et al. Quantitative analysis of the olfactory pathway for drug delivery to the brain. Brain Res 1995;692(1–2):278–82.

41. Born J, Lange T, Kern W, et al. Sniffing neuropeptides: a transnasal approach to the human brain. Nat Neurosci 2002;5(6):514–6.

42. Schulz C, Paulus K, Johren O, et al. Intranasal leptin reduces appetite and induces weight loss in rats with diet-induced obesity (DIO). Endocrinology 2012;153(1):143–53.

43. Schulz C, Paulus K, Lehnert H. Central nervous and metabolic effects of intranasally applied leptin. Endocrinology 2004;145(6):2696–701.

44. Shimizu H, Oh IS, Okada S, et al. Inhibition of appetite by nasal leptin administration in rats. Int J Obes 2005;29(7):858–63.

45. Degerman E, Landström TR, Holst LS, et al. Role for phosphodiesterase 3b in regulation of lipolysis and insulin secretion. In: LeRoith D, Olefsky JM, Taylor SI, editors. Diabetes mellitus: a fundamental and clinical text. 3rd edition. Philadelphia: Lippincott Williams & Wilkins; 2003. p. 374–81.

46. Assimacopoulos-Jeannet F, Brichard S, Rencurel F, et al. In vivo effects of hyperinsulinemia on lipogenic enzymes and glucose transporter expression in rat liver and adipose tissues. Metabolism 1995;44(2):228–33.

47. Grefhorst A, Hoekstra J, Derks TG, et al. Acute hepatic steatosis in mice by blocking beta-oxidation does not reduce insulin sensitivity of very-low-density lipoprotein production. Am J Physiol Gastrointest Liver Physiol 2005;289(3):G592–8.

48. Buettner C, Camacho RC. Hypothalamic control of hepatic glucose production and its potential role in insulin resistance. Endocrinol Metab Clin North Am 2008; 37(4):825–40.

49. Pocai A, Lam TK, Gutierrez-Juarez R, et al. Hypothalamic K(ATP) channels control hepatic glucose production. Nature 2005;434(7036):1026–31.

50. Okamoto H, Obici S, Accili D, et al. Restoration of liver insulin signaling in Insr knockout mice fails to normalize hepatic insulin action. J Clin Invest 2005; 115(5):1314–22.

51. Ramnanan CJ, Saraswathi V, Smith MS, et al. Brain insulin action augments hepatic glycogen synthesis without suppressing glucose production or gluconeogenesis in dogs. J Clin Invest 2011;121(9):3713–23.

52. Konner AC, Janoschek R, Plum L, et al. Insulin action in AgRP-expressing neurons is required for suppression of hepatic glucose production. Cell Metab 2007;5(6):438–49.

53. Ramnanan CJ, Edgerton DS, Cherrington AD. Evidence against a physiologic role for acute changes in CNS insulin action in the rapid regulation of hepatic glucose production. Cell Metab 2012;15(5):656–64.

54. Kishore P, Boucai L, Zhang K, et al. Activation of K(ATP) channels suppresses glucose production in humans. J Clin Invest 2011;121(12):4916–20.

55. Heni M, Kullmann S, Ketterer C, et al. Nasal insulin changes peripheral insulin sensitivity simultaneously with altered activity in homeostatic and reward-related human brain regions. Diabetologia 2012;55(6):1773–82.

56. Stockhorst U, de Fries D, Steingrueber HJ, et al. Unconditioned and conditioned effects of intranasally administered insulin vs placebo in healthy men: a randomised controlled trial. Diabetologia 2011;54(6):1502–6.

57. Benedict C, Brede S, Schioth HB, et al. Intranasal insulin enhances postprandial thermogenesis and lowers postprandial serum insulin levels in healthy men. Diabetes 2010;60(1):114–8.

58. Jauch-Chara K, Friedrich A, Rezmer M, et al. Intranasal insulin suppresses food intake via enhancement of brain energy levels in humans. Diabetes 2012;61(9): 2261–8.

59. Benedict C, Dodt C, Hallschmid M, et al. Immediate but not long-term intranasal administration of insulin raises blood pressure in human beings. Metabolism 2005;54(10):1356–61.

60. Clegg DJ, Riedy CA, Smith KA, et al. Differential sensitivity to central leptin and insulin in male and female rats. Diabetes 2003;52(3):682–7.

61. McGowan MK, Andrews KM, Grossman SP. Chronic intrahypothalamic infusions of insulin or insulin antibodies alter body weight and food intake in the rat. Physiol Behav 1992;51(4):753–66.

62. Brief DJ, Davis JD. Reduction of food intake and body weight by chronic intraventricular insulin infusion. Brain Res Bull 1984;12(5):571–5.

63. Menendez JA, Atrens DM. Insulin and the paraventricular hypothalamus: modulation of energy balance. Brain Res 1991;555(2):193–201.

64. Rahmouni K, Morgan DA, Morgan GM, et al. Hypothalamic PI3K and MAPK differentially mediate regional sympathetic activation to insulin. J Clin Invest 2004;114(5):652–8.

65. Benedict C, Kern W, Schultes B, et al. Differential sensitivity of men and women to anorexigenic and memory-improving effects of intranasal insulin. J Clin Endocrinol Metab 2008;93(4):1339–44.

66. Hallschmid M, Benedict C, Schultes B, et al. Intranasal insulin reduces body fat in men but not in women. Diabetes 2004;53(11):3024–9.

67. Guthoff M, Grichisch Y, Canova C, et al. Insulin modulates food-related activity in the central nervous system. J Clin Endocrinol Metab 2010;95(2):748–55.

68. Hallschmid M, Higgs S, Thienel M, et al. Postprandial administration of intranasal insulin intensifies satiety and reduces intake of palatable snacks in women. Diabetes 2012;61(4):782–9.

69. Higgs S, Williamson AC, Attwood AS. Recall of recent lunch and its effect on subsequent snack intake. Physiol Behav 2008;94(3):454–62.

70. Higgs S, Williamson AC, Rotshtein P, et al. Sensory-specific satiety is intact in amnesics who eat multiple meals. Psychol Sci 2008;19(7):623–8.

71. Rozin P, Dow S, Moscovitch M, et al. What causes humans to begin and end a meal? A role for memory for what has been eaten, as evidenced by a study of multiple meal eating in amnesic patients. Psychol Sci 1998;9(5):392–6.

72. Diekelmann S, Born J. The memory function of sleep. Nat Rev Neurosci 2010; 11(2):114–26.

73. Moult PR, Harvey J. Hormonal regulation of hippocampal dendritic morphology and synaptic plasticity. Cell Adh Migr 2008;2(4):269–75.

74. Craft S, Watson GS. Insulin and neurodegenerative disease: shared and specific mechanisms. Lancet Neurol 2004;3(3):169–78.

75. Seaquist ER, Damberg GS, Tkac I, et al. The effect of insulin on in vivo cerebral glucose concentrations and rates of glucose transport/metabolism in humans. Diabetes 2001;50(10):2203–9.

76. Hasselbalch SG, Knudsen GM, Videbaek C, et al. No effect of insulin on glucose blood-brain barrier transport and cerebral metabolism in humans. Diabetes 1999;48(10):1915–21.

77. Doyle P, Cusin I, Rohner-Jeanrenaud F, et al. Four-day hyperinsulinemia in euglycemic conditions alters local cerebral glucose utilization in specific brain nuclei of freely moving rats. Brain Res 1995;684(1):47–55.

78. Benedict C, Hallschmid M, Schmitz K, et al. Intranasal insulin improves memory in humans: superiority of insulin aspart. Neuropsychopharmacology 2007;32(1):239–43.

79. Reger MA, Watson GS, Green PS, et al. Intranasal insulin improves cognition and modulates beta-amyloid in early AD. Neurology 2008;70(6):440–8.

80. Reger MA, Watson GS, Green PS, et al. Intranasal insulin administration dose-dependently modulates verbal memory and plasma amyloid-beta in memory-impaired older adults. J Alzheimers Dis 2008;13(3):323–31.

81. Craft S, Baker LD, Montine TJ, et al. Intranasal insulin therapy for Alzheimer disease and amnestic mild cognitive impairment: a pilot clinical trial. Arch Neurol 2012;69(1):29–38.
82. Grillo CA, Piroli GG, Kaigler KF, et al. Downregulation of hypothalamic insulin receptor expression elicits depressive-like behaviors in rats. Behav Brain Res 2011;222(1):230–5.
83. Tschritter O, Preissl H, Hennige AM, et al. The cerebrocortical response to hyperinsulinemia is reduced in overweight humans: a magnetoencephalographic study. Proc Natl Acad Sci U S A 2006;103(32):12103–8.
84. Hallschmid M, Benedict C, Schultes B, et al. Obese men respond to cognitive but not to catabolic brain insulin signaling. Int J Obes (Lond) 2008;32(2):275–82.
85. Wang J, Obici S, Morgan K, et al. Overfeeding rapidly induces leptin and insulin resistance. Diabetes 2001;50(12):2786–91.
86. Ono H, Pocai A, Wang Y, et al. Activation of hypothalamic S6 kinase mediates diet-induced hepatic insulin resistance in rats. J Clin Invest 2008;118(8):2959–68.
87. Scherer T, Lindtner C, Zielinski E, et al. Short-term voluntary overfeeding disrupts brain insulin control of adipose tissue lipolysis. J Biol Chem 2012;287(39):33061–9.
88. Cornier MA, Bergman BC, Bessesen DH. The effects of short-term overfeeding on insulin action in lean and reduced-obese individuals. Metabolism 2006;55(9): 1207–14.
89. Brons C, Jensen CB, Storgaard H, et al. Impact of short-term high-fat feeding on glucose and insulin metabolism in young healthy men. J Physiol 2009;587(Pt 10): 2387–97.
90. Thaler JP, Yi CX, Schur EA, et al. Obesity is associated with hypothalamic injury in rodents and humans. J Clin Invest 2012;122(1):153–62.
91. Zhang X, Zhang G, Zhang H, et al. Hypothalamic IKKbeta/NF-kappaB and ER stress link overnutrition to energy imbalance and obesity. Cell 2008;135(1):61–73.
92. McCrimmon RJ, Ryan CM, Frier BM. Diabetes and cognitive dysfunction. Lancet 2012;379(9833):2291–9.
93. Gold SM, Dziobek I, Sweat V, et al. Hippocampal damage and memory impairments as possible early brain complications of type 2 diabetes. Diabetologia 2007;50(4):711–9.
94. Kodl CT, Seaquist ER. Cognitive dysfunction and diabetes mellitus. Endocr Rev 2008;29(4):494–511.
95. Tschritter O, Preissl H, Hennige AM, et al. High cerebral insulin sensitivity is associated with loss of body fat during lifestyle intervention. Diabetologia 2012;55(1):175–82.
96. Scherer T, Buettner C. Yin and Yang of hypothalamic insulin and leptin signaling in regulating white adipose tissue metabolism. Rev Endocr Metab Disord 2011; 12(3):235–43.
97. Gutierrez-Juarez R, Obici S, Rossetti L. Melanocortin-independent effects of leptin on hepatic glucose fluxes. J Biol Chem 2004;279(48):49704–15.
98. de Luca C, Kowalski TJ, Zhang Y, et al. Complete rescue of obesity, diabetes, and infertility in db/db mice by neuron-specific LEPR-B transgenes. J Clin Invest 2005;115(12):3484–93.
99. Guo K, McMinn JE, Ludwig T, et al. Disruption of peripheral leptin signaling in mice results in hyperleptinemia without associated metabolic abnormalities. Endocrinology 2007;148(8):3987–97.
100. Baicy K, London ED, Monterosso J, et al. Leptin replacement alters brain response to food cues in genetically leptin-deficient adults. Proc Natl Acad Sci U S A 2007;104(46):18276–9.

101. DelParigi A, Chen K, Salbe AD, et al. Successful dieters have increased neural activity in cortical areas involved in the control of behavior. Int J Obes 2007;31(3):440–8.

102. Farooqi IS, Bullmore E, Keogh J, et al. Leptin regulates striatal regions and human eating behavior. Science 2007;317(5843):1355.

103. Tataranni PA, Gautier JF, Chen K, et al. Neuroanatomical correlates of hunger and satiation in humans using positron emission tomography. Proc Natl Acad Sci U S A 1999;96(8):4569–74.

104. Scarpace PJ, Matheny M, Pollock BH, et al. Leptin increases uncoupling protein expression and energy expenditure. Am J Physiol 1997;273(1 Pt 1):E226–30.

105. Ahima RS, Prabakaran D, Mantzoros C, et al. Role of leptin in the neuroendocrine response to fasting. Nature 1996;382(6588):250–2.

106. Rosenbaum M, Nicolson M, Hirsch J, et al. Effects of weight change on plasma leptin concentrations and energy expenditure. J Clin Endocrinol Metab 1997; 82(11):3647–54.

107. Rosenbaum M, Goldsmith R, Bloomfield D, et al. Low-dose leptin reverses skeletal muscle, autonomic, and neuroendocrine adaptations to maintenance of reduced weight. J Clin Invest 2005;115(12):3579–86.

108. Sumithran P, Prendergast LA, Delbridge E, et al. Long-term persistence of hormonal adaptations to weight loss. N Engl J Med 2011;365(17):1597–604.

109. Leibel RL, Rosenbaum M, Hirsch J. Changes in energy expenditure resulting from altered body weight. N Engl J Med 1995;332(10):621–8.

110. Rosenbaum M, Sy M, Pavlovich K, et al. Leptin reverses weight loss-induced changes in regional neural activity responses to visual food stimuli. J Clin Invest 2008;118(7):2583–91.

111. Koyama K, Chen G, Wang MY, et al. beta-cell function in normal rats made chronically hyperleptinemic by adenovirus-leptin gene therapy. Diabetes 1997;46(8):1276–80.

112. Rossetti L, Massillon D, Barzilai N, et al. Short term effects of leptin on hepatic gluconeogenesis and in vivo insulin action. J Biol Chem 1997;272(44):27758–63.

113. Chinookoswong N, Wang JL, Shi ZQ. Leptin restores euglycemia and normalizes glucose turnover in insulin-deficient diabetes in the rat. Diabetes 1999; 48(7):1487–92.

114. Yu X, Park BH, Wang MY, et al. Making insulin-deficient type 1 diabetic rodents thrive without insulin. Proc Natl Acad Sci U S A 2008;105(37):14070–5.

115. Wang MY, Chen L, Clark GO, et al. Leptin therapy in insulin-deficient type I diabetes. Proc Natl Acad Sci U S A 2010;107(11):4813–9.

116. Hidaka S, Yoshimatsu H, Kondou S, et al. Chronic central leptin infusion restores hyperglycemia independent of food intake and insulin level in streptozotocin-induced diabetic rats. FASEB J 2002;16(6):509–18.

117. Lin CY, Higginbotham DA, Judd RL, et al. Central leptin increases insulin sensitivity in streptozotocin-induced diabetic rats. Am J Physiol Endocrinol Metab 2002;282(5):E1084–91.

118. Fujikawa T, Chuang JC, Sakata I, et al. Leptin therapy improves insulin-deficient type 1 diabetes by CNS-dependent mechanisms in mice. Proc Natl Acad Sci U S A 2010;107(40):17391–6.

119. Denroche HC, Levi J, Wideman RD, et al. Leptin therapy reverses hyperglycemia in mice with streptozotocin-induced diabetes, independent of hepatic leptin signaling. Diabetes 2011;60(5):1414–23.

120. Mittendorfer B, Horowitz JF, DePaoli AM, et al. Recombinant human leptin treatment does not improve insulin action in obese subjects with type 2 diabetes. Diabetes 2011;60(5):1474–7.

121. Moon HS, Matarese G, Brennan AM, et al. Efficacy of metreleptin in obese patients with type 2 diabetes: cellular and molecular pathways underlying leptin tolerance. Diabetes 2011;60(6):1647–56.
122. Mantzoros CS, Magkos F, Brinkoetter M, et al. Leptin in human physiology and pathophysiology. Am J Physiol Endocrinol Metab 2011;301(4):E567–84.
123. Szczepaniak LS, Nurenberg P, Leonard D, et al. Magnetic resonance spectroscopy to measure hepatic triglyceride content: prevalence of hepatic steatosis in the general population. Am J Physiol Endocrinol Metab 2005;288(2):E462–8.
124. Warne JP, Alemi F, Reed AS, et al. Impairment of central leptin-mediated PI3K signaling manifested as hepatic steatosis independent of hyperphagia and obesity. Cell Metab 2011;14(6):791–803.
125. Singh A, Wirtz M, Parker N, et al. Leptin-mediated changes in hepatic mitochondrial metabolism, structure, and protein levels. Proc Natl Acad Sci U S A 2009; 106(31):13100–5.
126. Cohen P, Zhao C, Cai X, et al. Selective deletion of leptin receptor in neurons leads to obesity. J Clin Invest 2001;108(8):1113–21.
127. Petersen KF, Oral EA, Dufour S, et al. Leptin reverses insulin resistance and hepatic steatosis in patients with severe lipodystrophy. J Clin Invest 2002; 109(10):1345–50.
128. Ebihara K, Kusakabe T, Hirata M, et al. Efficacy and safety of leptin-replacement therapy and possible mechanisms of leptin actions in patients with generalized lipodystrophy. J Clin Endocrinol Metab 2007;92(2):532–41.
129. Heymsfield SB, Greenberg AS, Fujioka K, et al. Recombinant leptin for weight loss in obese and lean adults: a randomized, controlled, dose-escalation trial. JAMA 1999;282(16):1568–75.
130. Pocai A, Morgan K, Buettner C, et al. Central leptin acutely reverses diet-induced hepatic insulin resistance. Diabetes 2005;54(11):3182–9.
131. El-Haschimi K, Pierroz DD, Hileman SM, et al. Two defects contribute to hypothalamic leptin resistance in mice with diet-induced obesity. J Clin Invest 2000;105(12):1827–32.
132. Banks WA, DiPalma CR, Farrell CL. Impaired transport of leptin across the blood-brain barrier in obesity. Peptides 1999;20(11):1341–5.
133. Burguera B, Couce ME, Curran GL, et al. Obesity is associated with a decreased leptin transport across the blood-brain barrier in rats. Diabetes 2000;49(7): 1219–23.
134. Ceccarini G, Flavell RR, Butelman ER, et al. PET imaging of leptin biodistribution and metabolism in rodents and primates. Cell Metab 2009;10(2):148–59.
135. Fliedner S, Schulz C, Lehnert H. Brain uptake of intranasally applied radioiodinated leptin in Wistar rats. Endocrinology 2006;147(5):2088–94.
136. Kern W, Benedict C, Schultes B, et al. Low cerebrospinal fluid insulin levels in obese humans. Diabetologia 2006;49(11):2790–2.
137. Fishel MA, Watson GS, Montine TJ, et al. Hyperinsulinemia provokes synchronous increases in central inflammation and beta-amyloid in normal adults. Arch Neurol 2005;62(10):1539–44.
138. Mayer CM, Belsham DD. Central insulin signaling is attenuated by long-term insulin exposure via insulin receptor substrate-1 serine phosphorylation, proteasomal degradation, and lysosomal insulin receptor degradation. Endocrinology 2010;151(1):75–84.
139. Bohringer A, Schwabe L, Richter S, et al. Intranasal insulin attenuates the hypothalamic-pituitary-adrenal axis response to psychosocial stress. Psychoneuroendocrinology 2008;33(10):1394–400.

Integrating Metabolism and Longevity Through Insulin and IGF1 Signaling

Marianna Sadagurski, PhD, Morris F. White, PhD*

KEYWORDS

- Central nervous system • Insulin/IGF signaling • Life span • Neurodegeneration
- Metabolism • Aging • Energy balance • Glucose homeostasis

KEY POINTS

- The insulin pathway coordinates growth, development, metabolic homoeostasis, fertility and stress resistance, which ultimately influence life span.
- Work in flies, nematodes and mice indicate that excess insulin signaling damages cellular function and accelerates aging.
- Maintenance of the central nervous system (CNS) has particular importance for life span.
- Genetic manipulations of insulin/IGF1 signaling are beginning to reveal neuronal circuits which might resolve the central regulation of systemic metabolism from organism longevity.

INTRODUCTION

Insulin/IGF1 signaling has pleiotropic biological effects in virtually all tissues; however, the role of insulin/IGF1 signaling in peripheral tissues has been studied far more extensively than its role in the brain.[1] Reduced insulin signaling, usually called insulin resistance in clinical circles, has serious detrimental effects that usually lead to excess circulating insulin and life-threatening metabolic disorders, including type 2 diabetes and cardiovascular disease.[2] By comparison, genetic strategies to reduce insulin/IGF1 signaling in *Caenorhabditis elegans*, *Drosophila melanogaster*, and rodents has emerged as a reliable means of extending life span.[3–7] Understanding the relation between insulin resistance and reduced insulin/IGF signaling might provide important insights into the pathology of metabolic disease, its sequelae, and strategies for treatment.

Department of Endocrinology, Children's Hospital Boston, Howard Hughes Medical Institute, 300 Longwood Avenue, Boston, MA 02115, USA
* Corresponding author. Division of Endocrinology, Howard Hughes Medical Institute, Children's Hospital Boston, Harvard Medical School, Center for Life Sciences, 3 Blackfan Circle, Room 16020, Boston, MA 02115.
E-mail address: morris.white@childrens.harvard.edu

Endocrinol Metab Clin N Am 42 (2013) 127–148
http://dx.doi.org/10.1016/j.ecl.2012.11.008
0889-8529/13/$ – see front matter © 2013 Published by Elsevier Inc.

endo.theclinics.com

Life expectancy in the industrialized world increased dramatically during the first two-thirds of the past century, from approximately 48 years to about 70 years, largely as a result of better nutrition, modern sanitation, antibiotics and immunization, and science-based medical diagnosis and treatment. Now reaching old age in good health might involve a favorable balance between hundreds of disease-causing and longevity-promoting genes and environmental factors, including the negative consequences of modern lifestyles and reduced activity.[8–11]

Experiments with various long-lived animal models reveal general strategies to reduce the progression of age-related diseases and neuronal degeneration. In particular, insulin and IGF1 signaling have emerged as conserved mechanisms that regulate nutrient homeostasis, growth, and life span. But contrary to conventional clinical medicine, where increased insulin signaling is a universal goal in the treatment of metabolic disease associated with obesity, type 2 diabetes and trauma, reduced insulin/IGF signaling can extend the life span of experimental animals. Moreover, age-related diseases, including Alzheimer disease (AD) and Huntington disease (HD), might be inversely related to the strength of brain insulin-like signaling.[12–17]

Although reduced insulin/IGF1 signaling in the central nervous system (CNS) extends life span and delays neurodegeneration processes, central insulin is also known to promote neuronal survival and memory, energy homeostasis, and reproduction.[18–23] In this review, this complex biology is discussed with particular emphasis on insulin signaling as a central homeostatic signal with regard to energy and glucose homeostasis and its role in neurodegenerative diseases.

INSULIN-LIKE SIGNALING PATHWAY
Receptors

Insulin-like signaling is an inclusive term that includes 3 homologous receptors in mammals: 2 insulin receptor isoforms (InsRA and InsRB) and 1 receptor for IGF1 (IGF1R). By comparison, invertebrates express a single orthologous receptor that recognizes a broad array of insulin-like peptides that are differentially expressed throughout the organism.[24] In mammals, the InsRs and IGF1R are encoded by 2 distinct genes that generate homologous precursors that are processed into alpha- and beta-subunits that dimerize to form a ligand-regulated transmembrane receptor tyrosine kinase. InsRB has 12 additional amino acids at the carboxyl terminus of the α-subunit that are omitted from InsRA by alternative splicing of Exon-11.[25,26] The InsRA predominates in liver and adipose tissue where it binds insulin much more strongly than it binds the insulin-like growth factors (IGF1 and IGF2). Unlike liver and adipose tissue, most tissues express both InsRs and IGF1R, which form hybrid receptors with distinct insulin-binding characteristics.[27] Neurons express mainly InsRB and IGF1R, which can form InsRB•IGF1R hybrids that bind insulin and IGF1/2 with moderate affinity, revealing how insulin and IGF1/2 signaling might be integrated to play common and distinct functions in the CNS.

IRS → AKT Cascade

The InsRs and IGF1R phosphorylate tyrosine residues in cellular proteins, including the insulin receptor substrates Irs1 and 2.[1,28,29] IRS proteins are adapter molecules that link the InsR and IGF1R to common downstream signaling cascades and heterologous regulatory mechanisms (**Fig. 1**). IRS proteins are targeted to the activated receptors through an NH_2-terminal pleckstrin homology (PH) domain and a phosphotyrosine binding (PTB) domain.[1] During insulin and IGF1 stimulation, tyrosine residues in the COOH terminus are phosphorylated and bound to the SH2 domains in various signaling proteins (see **Fig. 1**).[30] The interaction between IRS1 and the 85-kDa regulatory subunit (p85) of the class 1A PI3K is key to insulin-mediated control of metabolism and other cellular processes.[1] In addition to Irs1 and Irs2, the insulin receptor phosphorylates other proteins on tyrosine residues, including Shc, APS, and SH2B, Gab1/2, Dock1/2 and Cbl, and mass spectrometry reveals nearly 100 other tyrosyl phosphorylated proteins in insulin-stimulated cells.[31] Moreover, quantitative interaction proteomics based on SILAC technology reveals many proteins that might interact with Irs1.[32] Although the role of each of these substrates and binding proteins merit attention, work with knockout mice reveals that many insulin responses, especially those that are associated with somatic growth, carbohydrate, lipid, and protein metabolism are regulated through Irs1-mediated and 2-mediated activation of the PI3K→Akt cascade.[33–35]

AKT→mTORC Cascade

The IRS1/2→PI3K→Akt1/2 cascade phosphorylates many proteins, including Tsc2 (activates mTorc1) and FoxO1 (inhibits its nuclear regulation of gene expression) (see **Fig. 1**).[1,36–38] The TOR kinase is a principle signaling component regulated by nutrients in all cells. In yeast, it is encoded by 2 homologous genes (TOR1 and TOR2). In mammals, a single mTOR kinase form 2 complexes called mTORC1 and mTORC2 due to its association with Raptor or Rictor, respectively.[39] mTORC1 promotes nutrient storage (protein and lipid synthesis) and inhibits autophagy.[36–38,40] mTORC2 plays a role in the organization of the actin cytoskeleton, phosphorylates the COOH terminal site in Akt, and is required for mTORC1 activation and inhibition of FoxO nuclear localization[41,42] (see **Fig. 1**). Inhibition of the TOR pathway extends life span in worms, flies, and mice.[43] Raptor and Rictor have both been linked to mammalian longevity,[44] and treatment with rapamycin, an inhibitor of the mTOR pathway, significantly increases mouse life span.[45]

AKT→FoxO Cascade

FoxO transcription factors (mainly Foxo1 and 3) have broad tissue-specific functions linking gene expression to environmental stress, including glucose depletion, hypoxia, oxidative stress, and DNA damage.[46] In the brain, FoxO1 is predominantly expressed in the striatum, dentate gyrus, and ventral hippocampus, and FoxO3 is in the cortex, cerebellum, and hippocampus.[47,48] When starvation or insulin resistance are especially severe and cellular energy is depleted (increasing $[NAD^+]/[NADH]$), Sirt1 (silent mating type information regulation 2 homolog/NAD-dependent deacetylase) deacetylates FoxO1, which might adapt it toward severe stress protection.[49] In contrast, while cellular energy is high (reducing the $[NAD+/NADH]$), Sirt1 is relatively less active and acetylated FoxO has less activity toward certain nuclear targets.[46,49,50] Whether FoxO has beneficial or detrimental effects depends strongly on the metabolic and tissue context. For example, FoxO ablation in the arcuate nucleus of the hypothalamus results in reduced food intake, leanness, improved hepatic glucose homeostasis, and increased sensitivity to insulin and leptin.[51] Hyperactivated FoxO contributes significantly to the negative effects of hepatic insulin resistance, whereas hyperactivated FoxO might mediate some of the beneficial effects of reduced insulin signaling during neurodegeneration. Regardless of this complexity, the activation of FoxO factors during acute starvation generally promotes mitochondrial function and life-sustaining metabolism under environmental or physiologic stress.[52,53] However, during chronic insulin resistance, long-term FoxO activity leads to genetic remodeling that can cause cellular damage, even during nutrient excess.

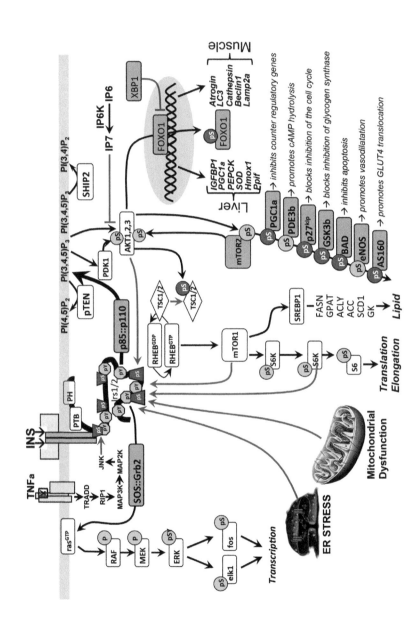

INSULIN/IGF1 SIGNALING IN THE CNS
Brain InsR and IGF1R Localization

InsR is generally abundant in neurons (cell bodies and synapses), but it is less abundant in glia. InsR is expressed in regions that are linked to olfaction, appetite, and autonomic functions, such as the olfactory bulb, limbic system, and hypothalamus, where it can influence feeding, body weight, and reproduction. InsR is also present in the choroid plexus, circumventricular organs, and brain microvessels,[54–56] suggesting it might contribute to the transport of insulin across the blood-brain barrier. IGF1R is expressed in the developing CNS and persists at high levels in the mature brain especially in the olfactory bulb, hippocampus, amygdala, parahippocampal gyrus, cerebellum, cortex, and caudate nucleus. IGF1R is less abundant in the substantia nigra, white matter and cerebral peduncles, and glia cells.[57–60]

Insulin/IGF1 in Brain Growth

Several mouse models demonstrate the importance of IGF1 signaling in brain growth and development.[61] Mice lacking IGF1 or IGF2 display a small brain. Most *IGF1*-null mice die perinatally, whereas others demonstrate uniform growth retardation up to 38%.[62,63] IGF2 is increased in *IGF1*-null mice suggesting that it might partially compensate for the loss of IGF1 expression.[64,65] Similarly, mice lacking *IGF1R* have smaller brains and die at birth.[66] Reduced brain size was also observed in transgenic mice over-expressing human IGFBP1 (IGF binding protein 1) in the brain or other organs as it blocks IGF1 binding to its receptor.[65] By contrast, neuron-specific disruption of the *InsR* gene (NIRKO mice) does not reduce brain size.[18] Glial cell activation showed no differences between NIRKO and control mice, suggesting that InsR is not required for neuronal survival *in vivo*. Conversely, whole-body or brain-specific *IRS2* deficiency uniformly reduces brain size between 30% and 40%.[6,67] Brains of the *IRS1*-null mice are only moderately smaller and proportional to the smaller body and cranial volume, similar to the effect of growth hormone receptor knockout.[68] Thus, the IGF1R→IRS2 pathway seems to play a crucial role in regulating neuronal growth and differentiation.

Brain Glucose Homeostasis

Insulin has dominant and well-characterized effects on glucose homeostasis in peripheral tissues; however, insulin also regulates glucose metabolism through specialized groups of glucose-sensing neurons in the arcuate nucleus of the hypothalamus. These neurons respond to peripheral signals to regulate feeding behavior and

◄──────

Fig. 1. A mechanism of insulin signaling. Insulin-regulated PI3K→PDK1→Akt and Grb2/Sos→ras kinase cascades. Insulin (INS) stimulates tyrosine phosphorylation of IRS proteins (pY), which promotes PI3K [p85•p110] and Grb2/SOS binding. Grb2/SOS stimulates the ras→MAPK (ERK1/2) cascade, which stimulates transcription factors. PI3K produces PI3,4P2 and PI3,4,5P3 (antagonized by the action of PTEN or SHIP2), which recruits PDK1 and AKT to the plasma membrane where AKT1 is activated by phosphorylation at T308 by PDK1 and S473 by mTORC2. AKT phosphorylates many cellular proteins including TSC2, which inhibits a Rheb-specific GTPase that activates mTORC1-dependent protein synthesis, and activation of SREBP1c, which stimulates lipogenic gene expression. AKT-mediated phosphorylation of FOXO1 results in cytoplasmic sequestration, which alters the expression of many genes in liver, muscle, brain, and other tissues. Akt, mTORC1, and S6K1 mediate homologous feedback inhibition of IRS-dependent signaling by Ser/Thr phosphorylation of IRS1/2, whereas circulating factors (TNFa) activate heterologous pathways that phosphorylate IRS on S/T sites.

energy homeostasis. These signals include the anorexigenic peptides proopiomelano-cortin (POMC) and cocaine-regulated and amphetamine-regulated transcript (CART), as well as the orexigenic neuropeptide Y (NPY) and agouti-related peptide (AgRP).[69,70] Under high glucose levels, brain insulin signaling hyperpolarizes glucose-sensing neurons to activate K^+/ATP channels and reduce neuronal firing (probably due to the inactivation of POMC neurons), which decreases body weight.[71] Conversely, impaired brain insulin signaling increases body weight.[18] This orexigenic effect is mediated by the activation of arcuate neurons containing NPY, AgRP, and γ-amino-butyric acid. Hypothalamic insulin also suppresses hepatic glucose production. Decreased hypothalamic insulin signaling reduces hepatic insulin sensitivity, which stimulates hepatic glucose production.[72] These results suggest that central insulin controls a hypothalamus → liver axis to regulate hepatic glucose production.[73,74]

Insulin/IGF1 Signaling in Neuronal Survival and Function

Insulin and IGF1 are neurotropic as they promote neuronal growth, survival, and differ-entiation under various experimental conditions, especially in the absence of other growth factors.[75,76] In the adult CNS, activation of the insulin/IGF1 signaling pathway by insulin and IGF1 is stimulatory to neuronal survival via the action of PI3K to directly inhibit apoptosis.[77] However, high levels of insulin in the brain are associated with neurotoxicity, which is believed to be due to increased production of free radicals and increased oxidative stress.[78] Insulin also induces neuronal cell death at physiolog-ically high concentrations in an in vitro rat hippocampal culture system.[79] IGF1 might inhibit neuronal survival by inhibiting SIRT1 expression: SIRT1 has been shown to have a protective effect on the survival of neuronal cells. The mechanism by which IGF1 regulates SIRT1 and its relevance to in vivo neuronal survival is as yet unknown.[80,81]

INVERTEBRATE INSULIN/IGF1 SIGNALING AND LIFE SPAN

At least 3 independent mechanisms regulate aging and life span, including caloric restriction, insulin/IGF signaling, and mitochondrial function.[82] The first studies demon-strating the involvement of the insulin-like pathway in the determination of life span came from C elegans.[83] An insulin-like signaling pathway in C elegans, consisting of proteins encoded by the genes daf-2, age-1, akt-1, akt-2, daf-16, and daf-18, regulates dauer diapause, reproduction, and life span.[84] Mutations that reduce the function of daf-2, age-1, or akt can increase the life span of C elegans.[83,85,86] These effects depend upon the presence of the dauer formation protein daf-16, an ortholog of mammalian FoxOs.[87] Inactivating mutations in daf-16 suppress the phenotype of the daf-2 or age-1 mutant.[88] Thus, insulin/IGFIR like signaling regulates aging by modulating gene expression.

In D melanogaster, a signaling pathway that includes the insulin/IGF1R, the insulin receptor substrate (CHICO), the PI3K (Dp110/p60), and the PI3K target PKB, regulates growth, size, and life span.[89] Mutation of the fly IR significantly extends life span.[90] Moreover, mutations of CHICO extend the life span of female flies by 48%.[91] Hetero-zygous deletion of the CHICO gene can increase life span, which is not further extended by calorie restriction. However, $CHICO^{+/-}$ flies are more easily starved by diluted food than are wild-type flies, whereas the maximal life span of $CHICO^{+/-}$ is less sensitive to reduction by high-energy food.[91] These results suggest that calorie restriction and reduced insulin-like signaling alter common downstream processes that extend life span. Regardless of the complexity, the informative genetic experi-ments with C elegans and flies provide a solid molecular basis to investigate the role of insulin signaling in the mammalian life span.

MAMMALIAN INSULIN/IGF1 SIGNALING AND LIFE SPAN
Endocrine Regulation of Life Span by Insulin/IGF1 Signaling

In mammals, the first evidence that insulin/IGF1 signaling is related to life span came from experiments with Snell and Ames mice, naturally occurring loss-of-function mutations that cause dwarfism. Snell mice have mutations in pituitary factor 1 (PIT1) and Ames mice have a mutation in Prop-1 that is required for PIT1 expression.[92] Compared with control mice, the life spans of Snell and Ames mice can increase 20% to 50%, depending on genetic background and diet. These mice are deficient in serum growth hormone (GH), thyroid-stimulating hormone (TSH), and prolactin (PRL), and display low circulating concentrations of insulin and IGF1. The prolonged longevity of Ames and Snell dwarf mice is most likely due to GH deficiency, because comparable extension of life span was described in mice that cannot release GH in response to GH-releasing hormone due to a GH receptor/GH-binding protein knockout (*GHRKO*).[92,93] Ames dwarf, Snell dwarf, and *GHRKO* mice share many phenotypic and physiologic characteristics that can contribute to the extended longevity.[94] Moreover, the decrease in the IR → IRS → PI3K pathway in the Snell dwarf mouse suggests that decreased activity of the insulin/IGF1 pathway might contribute to the longevity of the PIT1 mutant.[95]

Insulin and IGF1 Receptors and Life Span

Similar to GHRKO mice, IGF1 receptor–deficient mice are born 50% smaller than normal littermates, and die after a few days due to developmental defects.[66] However, a moderate decrease in IGF1R levels can extend mouse longevity. The loss of 1 copy of the *Igf1r* gene increases the life span of female mice by 33% and male mice by 16%.[96] In contrast to the Ames and Snell dwarf mice, *Igf1r* heterozygous mice have no alteration in fertility. *Igf1r* heterozygous mice are more resistant to oxidative stress, suggesting a possible mechanism of their increased life span.[96,97]

InsR-deficient mice die within a few days after birth due to severe hyperglycemia.[98] Mice retaining at least 20% of the normal InsR expression throughout the body can survive with severe postnatal growth retardation and hypoglycemia that resembles human leprechaunism.[99] This growth defect arises, at least in part, from increased hepatic IGFBP1, which reduces IGF1 bioavailability. Thus, small mice with severely reduced insulin or IGF1 signaling have short life spans as a result of developmental and metabolic defects. Whether the deletion of 1 allele of the InsR gene increases life span has not been investigated; however, as InsR$^{+/-}$ mice develop hyperinsulinemia, and 5% of them develop diabetes by 6 months of age, their statistical life span might be reduced.[100]

IRS Proteins and Life Span

IRS1 null mice are small and insulin resistant with nearly normal glucose homeostasis, due to β-cell expansion and compensatory hyperinsulinemia.[68] Some reports indicate a small increase in longevity of global *Irs1*$^{-/-}$ mice.[101] By contrast, global knockout IRS2 mice develop diabetes around 8 weeks of age, due to reduced β-cell mass and insufficient compensatory insulin secretion.[102,103] As a result of progressive diabetes, the life span of global *Irs2*$^{-/-}$ mice is reduced to about 15 weeks. Mice without *Irs2* and only a single allele of *Irs1* (*Irs1*$^{+/-}$•*Irs2*$^{-/-}$) develop severe fasting hyperglycemia and die by 4 weeks of age.[104] By contrast, mice retaining 1 allele of *Irs2* (*Irs1*$^{-/-}$•*Irs2*$^{+/-}$ mice) are small with nearly normal glucose tolerance and circulating insulin concentrations at 6 months of age[104]; however, these very small animals are fragile and require extraordinary care to live beyond this age. Thus, healthy glucose tolerance and a small size are not definitive determinants of life span.

Mutations in Insulin/IGF1 Signaling and Human Longevity

Several reports document a correlation between lower insulin/IGF1 activity and extreme human longevity.[105] Mutations in the *IGF1R* gene were found to be more abundant among Jewish Ashkenazi centenarians than in healthy controls.[106] Similarly, mutations within FoxO3a (the closest *daf-16* mammalian ortholog) correlate with the long-lived Japanese-Hawaiian or German centenarians.[107,108] In elderly women in the Leiden 85-plus study, polymorphisms of several genes related to insulin and somatotropic signaling were associated with reduced mortality and improved cognitive function.[109] IRS2 variants were also reported to correlate with longevity in an Italian population.[110] These studies support the hypothesis that subtle changes in insulin/IGF1 signaling might extend human life span. Regardless, insulin resistance in humans is ordinarily associated with life threatening metabolic disease.

INSULIN/IGF1 SIGNALING IN THE CNS: METABOLISM AND LIFE SPAN
Brain-Specific Inactivation of Insulin/IGF1 Signaling Molecules and Life Span Extension

Similar to whole-body heterozygous *IGF1R* mice,[96] brain-specific heterozygous *IGF1R*-knockout mice with genetically modified hyposensitivity for IGF1 in the CNS display increased life span.[111] By contrast, NIRKO mice (neuron-specific disruption of the InsR gene) display a normal life span. However, NIRKO mice display peripheral insulin resistance and obesity, but have normal brain development and neuronal survival.[18] A similar metabolic phenotype occurs in hypothalamic-specific *InsR* knockout mice.[112] In addition, drug-inducible, brain-specific, *InsR* knockout mice suffer from hyperinsulinemia and have an upregulation of hepatic leptin receptors.[72] The deletion of murine InsR from midbrain dopamine neurons causes hyperphagia and increased body weight.[113] These results demonstrate the importance of InsR in the CNS regulation of feeding and energy homeostasis.

Regulation of IRS2 signaling in the brain reveals a link between life span extension and metabolic regulation. Reduced IRS2 signaling in all tissues or just in the brain can increase the life span of mice maintained on a high-energy diet by nearly 6 months.[6] However, brain-specific, long-lived *IRS2* knockout mice consume approximately the same or slightly more food than the short-lived controls. At 22 months of age, brain *IRS2* knockout mice are overweight, hyperinsulinemic, and glucose intolerant.[6] Thus, less brain IRS2 signaling is associated with an increased life span regardless of the peripheral insulin sensitivity. The exact location of IRS2 signaling is important to investigate. Recent studies indicate that inhibiting IRS2 in the mouse midbrain attenuates the morphine reward.[114] Moreover, IRS2 in a subpopulation of hypothalamic neurons plays a role in energy homoeostasis and growth.[115] It is possible that the impact of altered insulin/IGF1 signaling in the brain on aging and metabolism will prove to be related to its action in a specific site or set of neurons.

Targeting Nutrient-Sensing Neural Circuits

The role of insulin-like signaling has focused on distinct populations of neurons in the hypothalamic arcuate nucleus (ArcN) that express POMC or AgRP; however, deletion of IRS2 or InsR from these neurons in mice has a negligible effect on metabolic homeostasis.[115–117] Similarly, disruption of the PI3K/Akt→FoxO1 pathway in POMC and AgRP neurons produces relatively subtle alterations in energy balance and glucose homeostasis.[118–120] Although insulin signaling in tyrosine hydroxylase (TH)-expressing catecholaminergic neurons is important for the control of mesolimbic dopamine (DA) signaling, lack of InsR signaling in these neurons has no effect on peripheral adiposity or glucose homeostasis.[113] By comparison, deletion of the InsR from steroidogenic factor 1 (SF1) neurons, a specific set of neurons of the ventrome-dial hypothalamus (VMH), promotes modest weight gain on a high-fat diet without altering energy balance or insulin sensitivity in chow-fed animals.[121] Thus, the relevant site at which insulin signaling contributes to metabolic regulation must be a distinct, or broader, set of neurons.

Although the mammalian CNS is far more complicated than that of worms and flies, recent advances provide insight into the neural circuitry that controls metabolism in mammals.[69] The peripheral hormone leptin signals the status of body energy stores to the CNS by binding and activating the leptin receptor (LepRb) on neurons that control energy balance and metabolism.[122] The dysregulation of all aspects of metab-olism, from glucose and lipid homeostasis to energy balance, in humans and rodents null for leptin or LepRb reflect the centrality of leptin → LepRb signaling to the regula-tion of metabolism.[123,124] LepRb neurons include those that express AgRP (as well as subsets of POMC, SF-1, and TH neurons) but also include other metabolically impor-tant neurons in the ARC and elsewhere.[70] Recently, it has been demonstrated that LepRb neurons represent the crucial mediators of brain insulin/IGF1 signaling in the control of energy balance and glucose homeostasis.[125] Thus, deletion of IRS2 from this restricted subset of CNS neurons dysregulates gene expression within the hypo-thalamic melanocortin system, which increases feeding, decreases energy expendi-ture, and promotes insulin resistance. This crucial set of neurons, which mediates the metabolic effects of IRS2 signaling in the brain, is by definition the same one that mediates leptin action, but IRS2 was not required for leptin action. Furthermore, although interference with leptin action in these LepRb neurons promotes reproduc-tive dysfunction, obesity and insulin resistance,[123] deletion of IRS2 and interference with insulin/IGF1 signaling in LepRb neurons does not alter the thyroid, adrenal, or reproductive axes.[125] Although leptin can promote some IRS2 → PI3K signaling,[126] leptin barely stimulates this pathway by comparison with insulin, suggesting that IRS2 functions primarily to mediate insulin/IGF1 rather than LepRb signaling in these neurons. Although the hypothalamic application of PI3K inhibitors or the genetic blockade of PI3K in some leptin responsive neurons impairs the acute anorectic response to leptin, these manipulations have little effect on baseline leptin action or energy balance.[71,126,127] Thus, although IRS2 signaling in LepRb neurons modulates metabolism, it does not seem to interact directly with leptin signaling.

Attenuation of the insulin/IGF1 pathway via IRS2 signaling in these nutrient-sensing leptin receptor–expressing neurons had no effect on IRS2-associated increase in life span (Sadagurski M, Dong X, Miller RA, Myers MG, White MF, unpublished data, 2012.). These results dissect the set of LepRb neurons that are responsible for the metabolic effects of insulin/IGF1 signaling in the CNS from yet unidentified neuronal circuits that underlie mammalian life span extension due to altered insulin/IGF1 signaling. Additional work will reveal new strategies to extend life span without causing undesirable metabolic side effects.

INSULIN/IGF1 SIGNALING AND NEURODEGENERATIVE DISEASES
Link Between Insulin/IGF1 Signaling and Neurodegeneration

Neurodegenerative diseases, including Alzheimer disease (AD), Parkinson disease (PD), and Huntington disease (HD), are associated with advanced age.[128–130] Most cases of AD and PD occur sporadically, and not earlier than the seventh decade of life. HD is a familial, monogenic disease that presents in middle age.[130] The adult onset of these neurodegenerative diseases might be related to progressive metabolic stress of aging. In humans, aging is associated with a decline in plasma levels of IGF1, which is suggested to contribute to disease progression.[131] By contrast, plasma insulin levels tend to increase with age, due to peripheral insulin resistance associated with weight gain and inactivity. Although the molecular link is controversial, neurodegeneration might be exacerbated by hyperinsulinemia and reduced peripheral IGF1.[33,78]

Studies on different invertebrate models suggest that genetic manipulations that reduce insulin-like signaling have the potential to reduce neurodegeneration and improve neuronal function with age.[24,132] In worms, long-lived *age-1* mutants show improved thermotaxis learning with age, which might be due to increased resistance to neuronal stresses and disease.[12,14] This protective effect was apparent in the worm model even when the alteration of insulin-like signaling was applied late in life.[14] In flies, the mutation *CHICO* slows age-related decline in motor function, suggesting that lowered insulin-like signaling has the potential to ameliorate CNS-based declines.[24,90]

Contemporary work suggests that it might be possible to slow the progression of neurodegeneration by modulating insulin-like signaling. Studies on rats demonstrate that infusion of IGF1 can protect against Aβ-mediated toxicity.[133] Injection of IGF1 into AD model mice reduces the typical behavioral impairments that are associated with increased amyloid-β (Aβ) levels.[134] Furthermore, IGF1 treatment of mouse primary neuronal cells transfected with mutant Huntington protein (HTT) inhibits polyQ-HTT aggregation and reduces cell death, presumably via the activation of the PI3K→AKT cascade.[135] In the cell-based functional genetic screen, increased expression of IRS2 led to a macroautophagy-mediated aggregate clearance of the accumulated HTT. However, the polyQ-toxicity protective effect was AKT independent, suggesting that unknown signals downstream of IRS2 diverge and more than 1 mechanism might be involved.[136]

These studies raise the possibility that insulin/IGF1 signaling might influence the progression of different stages of neurodegeneration. For example, hyperinsulinemia could exacerbate oxidative stress and the accumulation of damaged proteins, whereas reduced IGF1 might facilitate apoptosis and reduce the generation of new neurons.[82,137] However, increased peripheral signaling can attenuate the acute effects of insulin resistance and hyperglycemia. Thus, it remains controversial whether more or less insulin/IGF1 signaling can be expected to protect from progressive neurodegenerative disease.

Insulin/IGF1 Signaling in AD

AD is a chronic and progressive neurodegenerative disease and the most common form of dementia leading to the loss of cognitive abilities and death.[138] The disease is characterized by β-amyloid accumulation and the formation of extracellular amyloid plaques as well as neurofibrillary tangles. The β-amyloid plaques mainly contain aggregated Aβ peptides generated by proteolytic cleavage of the amyloid precursor protein (APP). The aggregation of Aβ is believed to be the principle cause of neurodegeneration in AD.[139] The removal or attenuated production of Aβ is an important clinical goal.

Recent studies suggest that CNS insulin resistance, sometimes called type 3 diabetes,[140] is associated with AD progression.[141] Two recent studies reveal an association between AD pathology and Ser/Thr phosphorylation (pS616[IRS1] and pS636[IRS1]/pS639[IRS1]) of IRS1. Phosphorylation at these sites has been found to be associated with reduced insulin sensitivity in cell culture experiments and in peripheral tissues.[142] Inflammation, excess nutrients, or chronic hyperinsulinemia are often linked to Ser/Thr phosphorylation of IRS1, so the exact profile of phosphorylation sites that accumulate might reveal the underlying cause of insulin resistance.[143,144] However, it is not clear what patterns of IRS1 Ser/Thr phosphorylation might reflect attenuated insulin/IGF1 signaling that contributes to disease pathology, or reflect a molecular counter-regulation to promote insulin/IGF signaling under stressful conditions.[143,144] For example, recent work suggests that Ser307, one of the principle phosphorylation sites on IRS1, might promote systemic insulin action (IRS1 tyrosine phosphorylation). In this scenario, Ser/Thr phosphorylation of IRS1 might be part of a mechanism to protect neurons by augmenting IGF signaling. It is also possible that reduced insulin signaling caused by Ser/Thr phosphorylation of IRS1 might protect neurons from proteotoxicity and decrease the Aβ load, in which case efforts to normalize Ser/Thr phosphorylation should be avoided.[15,16,145,146]

The Protective Effects of the Reduced Insulin/IGF1 Signaling in AD

Several studies have focused on the effects of reduced insulin/IGF1 signaling in AD mouse models.[15,16,145] The models include a transgenic mouse that accumulates Aβ plaques, due to the Swedish mutation (APP^{sw}) in APP (*Tg2576* mice). Intercrosses between *Tg2576* mice and mice lacking *IRS2* (*Tg2576•Irs2$^{-/-}$* mice) display a reduced Aβ plaque burden in the brain. Moreover, *Tg2576•Irs2$^{-/-}$* mice exhibit better learning and memory compared with *Tg2576* mice.[15] A similar study shows that female *Tg2576•Irs2$^{-/-}$* mice benefit most from the deletion of *IRS2*, because male mice develop early onset life-threatening diabetes due to the rapid and complete loss of beta cells. The deletion of *IGF1R* predominantly from the hippocampus of *Tg2576* mice by cre-recombinase under control of the synapsin-1 promoter (*Tg2576•nIGF1R$^{-/-}$*) protects both female and male mice against APP^{sw}-induced lethality.[16] Furthermore, the reduction in Aβ was observed specifically in hippocampus, but not in other brain regions. These results suggest an important role for the neuron-autonomous IGF1R→IRS2 pathway in the hippocampus in the control of APP metabolism.

Mice harboring only 1 copy of the IGF1R gene were also crossed to transgenic AD mice. These mice were protected from AD-associated memory and orientation impairments and had reduced rates of neuro-inflammation, and neuronal and synaptic losses in the aged brain. Due to the appearance of smaller and highly dense Aβ plaques, it is suggested that reduced IGF1 signaling protects the brain by sequestering highly toxic Aβ oligomers.[145] Although no data were reported on the metabolic status of these animals, based on the phenotype of the *IGF1R* heterozygous mice, it is reasonable to assume that glucose metabolism was not affected in these animals.

The Protective Effects of Reduced Insulin/IGF1 Signaling in the Mouse Model of HD

Compared with the lengthy degenerative processes associated with mortality in AD, neurodegeneration in HD progresses predictably to death depending on the length of an expanded CAG triplet repeat in the HD gene that encodes a mutant form of the HTT.[147] Mutant HTT produces intranuclear and cytoplasmic inclusions and kills cells in the striatum and cerebral cortex, although other areas are also affected.[148] We investigated the relation between IRS2 signaling and the progression of HD in R6/2 mice.[17] R6/2 mice were selected because they display a rapid and highly reproducible phenotype of neurodegeneration and are used frequently as a model of HD.[149] We hypothesized that HD might represent a suitable model to examine the effects of IRS2 signaling on degenerative processes in the CNS. Two experiments show that the levels of IRS2 signaling can modulate HD progression in R6/2 mice. Increasing IRS2 levels by 50% with a neuron-specific enolase transgene (*R6/2•Irs2^{ntg}*) accelerates the progression of neurodegeneration and significantly reduces the life span of R6/2 mice. In contrast, reducing IRS2 levels throughout the body, except in β cells where IRS2 expression is needed to prevent diabetes onset, extends the life span of R6/2 mice.[17] These results are consistent with the hypothesis that reduced IRS2 signaling (insulin/IGF1 resistance) might be protective against the effects of proteotoxicity.

PolyQ-HTT causes pathologic sequelae in R6/2 mice that develop progressively until death, including mitochondrial dysfunction and oxidative stress, accumulation of protein aggregates in the CNS, neuroinflammation, and abnormal behavior and movement.[149–151] However, only mitochondrial dysfunction and oxidative stress increase significantly in the CNS of $R6/2 \bullet Irs2^{ntg}$ mice, revealing a major consequence of excess insulin/IGF signaling on acute neurodegeneration and early death of these HD mice.[17] The slower progression of HD-like symptoms in R6/2 mice with less IRS2 expression is associated with increased nuclear localization of the transcription factor FoxO1. Some FoxO1 target genes are expressed at higher levels in the CNS of these mutant mice, including Ppargc1α and SOD2, both of which have strong effects on energy homeostasis and prevention of oxidative stress.[152,153] Whether neuronal mitochondrial damage and oxidative stress during normal aging is modulated by IRS2 signaling is an interesting disease model to establish, as it might have broad consequences on the progression of debilitating disease in an aging population. Our previous work shows that less neuronal IRS2 signaling preserves a youthful diurnal transition between glucose and fat oxidation, which is ordinarily lost in old wild-type mice.[6] Thus, the negative effects of IRS2 signaling on energy homeostasis in HD mice might exacerbate a common mechanism that contributes to the slow progressive neurodegeneration of normal aging.

R6/2 mice with reduced IRS2 signaling accumulate fewer polyQ-HTT aggregates in the brain.[17] Aggregate accumulation is believed to reflect cellular damage, as cells that form aggregates earlier tend to die earlier.[154] Aggregates might impair mitochondrial oxidative phosphorylation and contribute to free radical damage[155]; however, other modes of protection, such as increased autophagy might facilitate the clearance of protein aggregates.[156] Autophagy sequesters damaged organelles, including soluble and aggregate forms of mutant HTT, into double-membrane structures (autophagosomes) for degradation.[156,157] Increased nuclear FoxO-mediated gene expression, due to less IRS2 signaling, might increase the expression of genes that mediate autophagy and promote autophagosomes formation. Thus, increased autophagy might be responsible for the reduced HTT aggregates and slower HD progression in mice with reduced IRS2 expression levels.

Mutant HTT leads to the dysregulation of several cellular pathways, including gene transcription, mitochondrial function, oxidative stress resistance, and protein degradation pathways.[147] Decreased IRS2 signaling slows the progression of several of these pathogenic abnormalities, which attenuates the disease phenotypes in R6/2 mice (**Fig. 2**). Our results suggest that attenuation of the insulin/IGF1 signaling cascade, as a regulator of multiple cellular pathways, can slow disease progression, and thus, represents a potential therapeutic strategy to optimize neuroprotection during progressive genetic stress. Although increasing insulin signaling in peripheral tissues might be necessary to avoid the consequences of peripheral metabolic disease (insulin resistance, dyslipidemia, and cardiovascular disease), it is equally important to appreciate the potential life-threatening consequences of increased insulin/IGF1 → IRS2 signaling in the brain.

Autophagy as a Therapeutic Target

What candidate mechanism can be a potential therapeutic target that will contribute to life span extension and neuronal survival due to reduced insulin/IGF1 signaling? One of the potential therapeutic targets is the autophagy mechanism.[158,159] Autophagy is

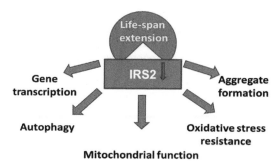

Fig. 2. Mechanisms regulated by reduced IRS2 levels to prevent HD progression. Decreased IRS2 signaling slows the progression of HD by manipulating several cellular pathways, including gene transcription, mitochondrial function, oxidative stress resistance, autophagy, and protein degradation pathways in R6/2 mice.

crucial for cell survival under extreme conditions, by removing damaged organelles and using the components for energy or repair. Autophagy might have a direct impact on reducing progressive aging, especially neurodegeneration.[159]

Autophagy was first associated with longevity because it is required for the life span extension of insulin-like signaling mutant worms.[160] Promoting autophagy in neurons is sufficient to extend life span and increase resistance to oxidative stress, possibly via the prevention of age-dependent accumulation of neuronal damage.[161–163] As autophagy is predominantly regulated by the TOR pathway, lowered insulin/IGF1 signaling might induce autophagy by attenuating the IRS → AKT → mTOR cascade.[164] Rapamycin is highly effective in inducing autophagy and reducing the load of misfolded proteins *in vitro* and in mouse models.[165] Thus, rapamycin or other mTORC1 inhibitors might serve to slow the accumulation of misfolded proteins.[166] However, the risk of diabetes due to rapamycin-induced suppression of insulin signaling components has diminished enthusiasm for its long-term use.[167]

The development of small molecules that can activate autophagy without cytotoxicity could emerge as a novel therapeutic approach to ameliorate brain pathologic conditions associated with aging. For example, psammaplysene A increases nuclear localization of FoxO3 *in vitro* and *in vivo*, which seems to protect motor neurons and fly eyes from toxic protein aggregation.[168] This study provides evidence that manipulating this longevity-promoting signaling pathway can effectively block neurodegeneration. Although it is not obvious how to modulate IRS2 signaling in specific neurons, compounds that reduce IRS2 levels in the brain without similar effects in peripheral tissues (especially pancreatic beta cells) would seem to be worth investigating. A strategy to reduce IRS2 signaling in a specific set of neurons might clear misfolded proteins to slow the progression of neurodegenerative diseases without undesirable peripheral metabolic effects.

FUTURE PERSPECTIVES

Although insulin and IGF signaling are well known for their system-wide effects on metabolism and organism growth, their effects on longevity might be nonautonomous and emanate from the CNS.[82,169] Although genetic manipulations to reduce insulin/IGF1 signaling in the mammalian CNS can extend longevity, they also cause peripheral insulin resistance and hyperglycemia, as in cases of long-lived brain-specific IGFR[+/−] mice and IRS2 brain-specific knockout mice.[6,111] However, with further analysis it might be possible to resolve the effects of insulin/IGF signaling on metabolism and life span. As the neuronal population that is responsible for the metabolic effects of insulin/IGF1 signaling pathway is unraveled, efforts can concentrate on identifying neural circuits that mediate the beneficial effects of reduced insulin/IGF1 signaling on life span and neurodegeneration while maintaining CNS energy homeostasis and peripheral glucose metabolism.

REFERENCES

1. White MF, Copps KD, Ozcan U, et al. The molecular basis of insulin action. In: Jameson JL, DeGroot LJ, editors. Endocrinology. 6th edition. Philadelphia: Elsevier; 2010. p. 636–59.
2. Bailey CJ. Treating insulin resistance: future prospects. Diab Vasc Dis Res 2007; 4(1):20–31.
3. Berman JR, Kenyon C. Germ-cell loss extends *C. elegans* life span through regulation of DAF-16 by kri-1 and lipophilic-hormone signaling. Cell 2006; 124(5):1055–68.
4. Guarente L, Ruvkun G, Amasino R. Aging, life span, and senescence. Proc Natl Acad Sci U S A 1998;95(19):11034–6.
5. Hertweck M, Gobel C, Baumeister R. *C. elegans* SGK-1 is the critical component in the Akt/PKB kinase complex to control stress response and life span. Dev Cell 2004;6(4):577–88.
6. Taguchi A, Wartschow LM, White MF. Brain IRS2 signaling coordinates life span and nutrient homeostasis. Science 2007;317(5836):369–72.
7. Wolf G. Calorie restriction increases life span: a molecular mechanism. Nutr Rev 2006;64(2 Pt 1):89–92.
8. Perls TT, Kunkel LM, Puca AA. The genetics of exceptional human longevity. J Am Geriatr Soc 2002;50(2):359–68.
9. Mattison JA, Roth GS, Beasley TM, et al. Impact of caloric restriction on health and survival in rhesus monkeys from the NIA study. Nature 2012;489(7415): 318–21.
10. Fraser HB, Khaitovich P, Plotkin JB, et al. Aging and gene expression in the primate brain. PLoS Biol 2005;3(9):e274.
11. Perls T, Kunkel LM, Puca A. The genetics of aging. Curr Opin Genet Dev 2002; 12(3):362–9.
12. Morley JF, Brignull HR, Weyers JJ, et al. The threshold for polyglutamine-expansion protein aggregation and cellular toxicity is dynamic and influenced by aging in *Caenorhabditis elegans*. Proc Natl Acad Sci U S A 2002;99(16): 10417–22.
13. Hsu AL, Murphy CT, Kenyon C. Regulation of aging and age-related disease by DAF-16 and heat-shock factor. Science 2003;300(5622):1142–5.
14. Cohen E, Bieschke J, Perciavalle RM, et al. Opposing activities protect against age-onset proteotoxicity. Science 2006;313(5793):1604–10.
15. Killick R, Scales G, Leroy K, et al. Deletion of Irs2 reduces amyloid deposition and rescues behavioural deficits in APP transgenic mice. Biochem Biophys Res Commun 2009;386(1):257–62.
16. Freude S, Hettich MM, Schumann C, et al. Neuronal IGF-1 resistance reduces Abeta accumulation and protects against premature death in a model of Alzheimer's disease. FASEB J 2009;23(10):3315–24.
17. Sadagurski M, Cheng Z, Rozzo A, et al. IRS2 increases mitochondrial dysfunction and oxidative stress in a mouse model of Huntington disease. J Clin Invest 2011;121(10):4070–81.

18. Bruning JC, Gautam D, Burks DJ, et al. Role of brain insulin receptor in control of body weight and reproduction. Science 2000;289(5487):2122–5.
19. Freude S, Schilbach K, Schubert M. The role of IGF-1 receptor and insulin receptor signaling for the pathogenesis of Alzheimer's disease: from model organisms to human disease. Curr Alzheimer Res 2009;6(3):213–23.
20. Plum L, Schubert M, Bruning JC. The role of insulin receptor signaling in the brain. Trends Endocrinol Metab 2005;16(2):59–65.
21. Schubert M, Gautam D, Surjo D, et al. Role for neuronal insulin resistance in neurodegenerative diseases. Proc Natl Acad Sci U S A 2004;101(9):3100–5.
22. Park CR, Seeley RJ, Craft S, et al. Intracerebroventricular insulin enhances memory in a passive-avoidance task. Physiol Behav 2000;68(4):509–14.
23. Craft S, Baker LD, Montine TJ, et al. Intranasal insulin therapy for Alzheimer disease and amnestic mild cognitive impairment: a pilot clinical trial. Arch Neurol 2012;69(1):29–38.
24. Partridge L, Gems D. The evolution of longevity. Curr Biol 2002;12(16):R544–6.
25. Ward CW, Garrett TP, McKern NM, et al. Structure of the insulin receptor family: unexpected relationships with other proteins. Today's Life Sciences 1999;11(2): 26–32.
26. Ward CW, Garrett TP. Structural relationships between the insulin receptor and epidermal growth factor receptor families and other proteins. Curr Opin Drug Discov Devel 2004;7(5):630–8.
27. Cheng Z, Tseng Y, White MF. Insulin signaling meets mitochondria in metabolism. Trends Endocrinol Metab 2010;21(10):589–98.
28. White MF, Maron R, Kahn CR. Insulin rapidly stimulates tyrosine phosphorylation of a Mr 185,000 protein in intact cells. Nature 1985;318:183–6.
29. Sun XJ, Rothenberg PL, Kahn CR, et al. The structure of the insulin receptor substrate IRS-1 defines a unique signal transduction protein. Nature 1991; 352:73–7.
30. White MF, Myers MG Jr. The molecular basis of insulin action. In: DeGroot LJ, Jameson JL, editors. Endocrinology. 4th edition. Philadelphia: WB Saunders; 2001. p. 712–27.
31. Schmelzle K, Kane S, Gridley S, et al. Temporal dynamics of tyrosine phosphorylation in insulin signaling. Diabetes 2006;55(8):2171–9.
32. Hanke S, Mann M. The phosphotyrosine interactome of the insulin receptor family and its substrates IRS-1 and IRS-2. Mol Cell Proteomics 2009;8(3):519–34.
33. White MF. Insulin signaling in health and disease. Science 2003;302(5651):1710–1.
34. Long YC, Cheng Z, Copps KD, et al. Insulin receptor substrates Irs1 and Irs2 coordinate skeletal muscle growth and metabolism via Akt and AMPK pathways. Mol Cell Biol 2011;31(3):430–41.
35. Guo S, Copps KD, Dong X, et al. The Irs1 branch of the insulin signaling cascade plays a dominant role in hepatic nutrient homeostasis. Mol Cell Biol 2009;29(18):5070–83.
36. Yecies JL, Zhang HH, Menon S, et al. Akt stimulates hepatic SREBP1c and lipogenesis through parallel mTORC1-dependent and independent pathways. Cell Metab 2011;14(1):21–32.
37. Wan M, Leavens KF, Saleh D, et al. Postprandial hepatic lipid metabolism requires signaling through Akt2 independent of the transcription factors FoxA2, FoxO1, and SREBP1c. Cell Metab 2011;14(4):516–27.
38. Hagiwara A, Cornu M, Cybulski N, et al. Hepatic mTORC2 activates glycolysis and lipogenesis through Akt, glucokinase, and SREBP1c. Cell Metab 2012; 15(5):725–38.

39. Kim DH, Sabatini DM. Raptor and mTOR: subunits of a nutrient-sensitive complex. Curr Top Microbiol Immunol 2004;279:259–70.
40. Laplante M, Sabatini DM. An emerging role of mTOR in lipid biosynthesis. Curr Biol 2009;19(22):R1046–52.
41. Zhang HH, Huang J, Duvel K, et al. Insulin stimulates adipogenesis through the Akt-TSC2-mTORC1 pathway. PLoS One 2009;4(7):e6189.
42. Jacinto E, Loewith R, Schmidt A, et al. Mammalian TOR complex 2 controls the actin cytoskeleton and is rapamycin insensitive. Nat Cell Biol 2004;6(11):1122–8.
43. Mouchiroud L, Molin L, Dalliere N, et al. Life span extension by resveratrol, rapamycin, and metformin: the promise of dietary restriction mimetics for an healthy aging. Biofactors 2010;36(5):377–82.
44. Sarbassov DD, Ali SM, Sabatini DM. Growing roles for the mTOR pathway. Curr Opin Cell Biol 2005;17(6):596–603.
45. Miller RA, Harrison DE, Astle CM, et al. Rapamycin, but not resveratrol or simvastatin, extends life span of genetically heterogeneous mice. J Gerontol A Biol Sci Med Sci 2011;66(2):191–201.
46. Salih DA, Brunet A. FoxO transcription factors in the maintenance of cellular homeostasis during aging. Curr Opin Cell Biol 2008;20(2):126–36.
47. Renault VM, Rafalski VA, Morgan AA, et al. FoxO3 regulates neural stem cell homeostasis. Cell Stem Cell 2009;5(5):527–39.
48. van der Horst A, Burgering BM. Stressing the role of FoxO proteins in lifespan and disease. Nat Rev Mol Cell Biol 2007;8(6):440–50.
49. Banks AS, Kim-Muller JY, Mastracci TL, et al. Dissociation of the glucose and lipid regulatory functions of FoxO1 by targeted knockin of acetylation-defective alleles in mice. Cell Metab 2011;14(5):587–97.
50. Kitamura YI, Kitamura T, Kruse JP, et al. FoxO1 protects against pancreatic beta cell failure through NeuroD and MafA induction. Cell Metab 2005;2(3): 153–63.
51. Ren H, Orozco IJ, Su Y, et al. FoxO1 target Gpr17 activates AgRP neurons to regulate food intake. Cell 2012;149(6):1314–26.
52. Cheng Z, White MF. Foxo1 in hepatic lipid metabolism. Cell Cycle 2010;9(2): 219–20.
53. Cheng Z, Guo S, Copps K, et al. Foxo1 integrates insulin signaling with mitochondrial function in the liver. Nat Med 2009;15(11):1307–11.
54. Gammeltoft S, Fehlmann M, Van Obberghen E. Insulin receptors in the mammalian central nervous system: binding characteristics and subunit structure. Biochimie 1985;67:1147–53.
55. Hill JM, Lesniak MA, Pert CB, et al. Autoradiographic localization of insulin receptors in rat brain: prominence in olfactory and limbic areas. Neuroscience 1986;17:1127–38.
56. Marks JL, Porte D Jr, Stahl WL, et al. Localization of insulin receptor mRNA in rat brain by in situ hybridization. Endocrinology 1990;127(6):3234–6.
57. Goodyer CG, De SL, Lai WH, et al. Characterization of insulin-like growth factor receptors in rat anterior pituitary, hypothalamus, and brain. Endocrinology 1984; 114(4):1187–95.
58. Joseph DA, Ye P. Expanding the mind: insulin-like growth factor I and brain development. Endocrinology 2008;149(12):5958–62.
59. Marks JL, Porte D Jr, Baskin DG. Localization of type I insulin-like growth factor receptor messenger RNA in the adult rat brain by in situ hybridization. Mol Endocrinol 1991;5(8):1158–68.

60. Bohannon NJ, Figlewicz DP, Corp ES, et al. Identification of binding sites for an insulin-like growth factor (IGF- I) in the median eminence of the rat brain by quantitative autoradiography. Endocrinology 1986;119(2):943–5.
61. Dupont J, Holzenberger M. Biology of insulin-like growth factors in development. Birth Defects Res C Embryo Today 2003;69(4):257–71.
62. Beck KD, Powell-Braxton L, Widmer HR, et al. IGF-1 gene disruption results in reduced brain size, CNS hypomyelination, and loss of hippocampal granule and striatal parvalbumin-containing neurons. Neuron 1995;14(4):717–30.
63. Nakae J, Kido Y, Accili D. Distinct and overlapping functions of insulin and IGF-I receptors. Endocr Rev 2001;22(6):818–35.
64. Ludwig T, Eggenschwiler J, Fisher P, et al. Mouse mutants lacking the type 2 IGF receptor (IGF2R) are rescued from perinatal lethality in Igf2 and Igf1r null backgrounds. Dev Biol 1996;177(2):517–35.
65. Butler AA, LeRoith D. Minireview: tissue-specific versus generalized gene targeting of the igf1 and igf1r genes and their roles in insulin-like growth factor physiology. Endocrinology 2001;142(5):1685–8.
66. Liu JP, Baker J, Perkins JA, et al. Mice carrying null mutations of the genes encoding insulin-like growth factor I (Igf-1) and type 1 IGF receptor (Igf1r). Cell 1993;75:59–72.
67. Schubert M, Brazil DP, Burks DJ, et al. Insulin receptor substrate-2 deficiency impairs brain growth and promotes tau phosphorylation. J Neurosci 2003; 23(18):7084–92.
68. Araki E, Lipes MA, Patti ME, et al. Alternative pathway of insulin signalling in mice with targeted disruption of the IRS-1 gene. Nature 1994;372(6502):186–90.
69. Leshan RL, Bjornholm M, Munzberg H, et al. Leptin receptor signaling and action in the central nervous system. Obesity (Silver Spring) 2006;14(Suppl 5): 208S–12S.
70. Myers MG Jr, Munzberg H, Leininger GM, et al. The geometry of leptin action in the brain: more complicated than a simple ARC. Cell Metab 2009;9(2):117–23.
71. Niswender KD, Morrison CD, Clegg DJ, et al. Insulin activation of phosphatidylinositol 3-kinase in the hypothalamic arcuate nucleus: a key mediator of insulin-induced anorexia. Diabetes 2003;52(2):227–31.
72. Koch L, Wunderlich FT, Seibler J, et al. Central insulin action regulates peripheral glucose and fat metabolism in mice. J Clin Invest 2008;118(6):2132–47.
73. Pocai A, Obici S, Schwartz GJ, et al. A brain-liver circuit regulates glucose homeostasis. Cell Metab 2005;1(1):53–61.
74. Plum L, Belgardt BF, Bruning JC. Central insulin action in energy and glucose homeostasis. J Clin Invest 2006;116(7):1761–6.
75. de la Monte SM, Tong M, Lester-Coll N, et al. Therapeutic rescue of neurodegeneration in experimental type 3 diabetes: relevance to Alzheimer's disease. J Alzheimers Dis 2006;10(1):89–109.
76. Russo VC, Gluckman PD, Feldman EL, et al. The insulin-like growth factor system and its pleiotropic functions in brain. Endocr Rev 2005;26(7):916–43.
77. Van Der Heide LP, Ramakers GM, Smidt MP. Insulin signaling in the central nervous system: learning to survive. Prog Neurobiol 2006;79(4):205–21.
78. Barbieri M, Rizzo MR, Manzella D, et al. Glucose regulation and oxidative stress in healthy centenarians. Exp Gerontol 2003;38(1–2):137–43.
79. Tanaka Y, Takata T, Satomi T, et al. The double-edged effect of insulin on the neuronal cell death associated with hypoglycemia on the hippocampal slice culture. Kobe J Med Sci 2008;54(2):E97–107.

80. Michan S, Sinclair D. Sirtuins in mammals: insights into their biological function. Biochem J 2007;404(1):1–13.
81. Cohen HY, Miller C, Bitterman KJ, et al. Calorie restriction promotes mammalian cell survival by inducing the SIRT1 deacetylase. Science 2004;305(5682): 390–2.
82. Taguchi A, White MF. Insulin-like signaling, nutrient homeostasis, and life span. Annu Rev Physiol 2008;70:191–212.
83. Morris JZ, Tissenbaum HA, Ruvkun G. A phosphatidylinositol-3-OH kinase family member regulating longevity and diapause in *Caenorhabditis elegans*. Nature 1996;382(6591):536–9.
84. Tissenbaum HA, Ruvkun G. An insulin-like signaling pathway affects both longevity and reproduction in *Caenorhabditis elegans*. Genetics 1998;148(2): 703–17.
85. Wolkow CA, Kimura KD, Lee MS, et al. Regulation of *C. elegans* life-span by insulinlike signaling in the nervous system. Science 2000;290(5489):147–50.
86. Kimura KD, Tissenbaum HA, Liu Y, et al. daf-2, an insulin receptor-like gene that regulates longevity and diapause in *Caenorhabditis elegans* [see comments]. Science 1997;277(5328):942–6.
87. Lin K, Dorman JB, Rodan A, et al. daf-16: an HNF-3/forkhead family member that can function to double the life-span of *Caenorhabditis elegans* [see comments]. Science 1997;278(5341):1319–22.
88. Ogg S, Paradis S, Gottlieb S, et al. The Fork head transcription factor DAF-16 transduces insulin-like metabolic and longevity signals in *C. elegans*. Nature 1997;389(6654):994–9.
89. Aigaki T, Seong KH, Matsuo T. Longevity determination genes in *Drosophila melanogaster*. Mech Ageing Dev 2002;123(12):1531–41.
90. Tatar M, Kopelman A, Epstein D, et al. A mutant *Drosophila* insulin receptor homolog that extends life-span and impairs neuroendocrine function. Science 2001;292(5514):107–10.
91. Clancy DJ, Gems D, Harshman LG, et al. Extension of life-span by loss of CHICO, a *Drosophila* insulin receptor substrate protein. Science 2001;292(5514):104–6.
92. Bartke A, Brown-Borg H. Life extension in the dwarf mouse. Curr Top Dev Biol 2004;63:189–225.
93. Steger RW, Bartke A, Cecim M. Premature ageing in transgenic mice expressing different growth hormone genes. J Reprod Fertil Suppl 1993;46:61–75.
94. Bartke A. Impact of reduced insulin-like growth factor-1/insulin signaling on aging in mammals: novel findings. Aging Cell 2008;7(3):285–90.
95. Hsieh CC, DeFord JH, Flurkey K, et al. Implications for the insulin signaling pathway in Snell dwarf mouse longevity: a similarity with the *C. elegans* longevity paradigm. Mech Ageing Dev 2002;123(9):1229–44.
96. Holzenberger M, Dupont J, Ducos B, et al. IGF-1 receptor regulates lifespan and resistance to oxidative stress in mice. Nature 2003;421(6919):182–7.
97. Holzenberger M. The role of insulin-like signalling in the regulation of ageing. Horm Res 2004;62(Suppl 1):89–92.
98. Accili D, Drago J, Lee EJ, et al. Early neonatal death in mice homozygous for a null allele of the insulin receptor gene. Nat Genet 1996;12(1):106–9.
99. Nandi A, Kitamura T, Kahn CR, et al. Mouse models of insulin resistance. Physiol Rev 2004;84(2):623–47.
100. Kido Y, Burks DJ, Withers D, et al. Tissue-specific insulin resistance in mice with mutations in the insulin receptor, IRS-1, and IRS-2. J Clin Invest 2000;105(2): 199–205.

101. Selman C, Lingard S, Choudhury AI, et al. Evidence for lifespan extension and delayed age-related biomarkers in insulin receptor substrate 1 null mice. FASEB J 2007;22(3):807–18.
102. Withers DJ, Gutierrez JS, Towery H, et al. Disruption of IRS-2 causes type 2 diabetes in mice. Nature 1998;391(6670):900–4.
103. Withers DJ, Burks DJ, Towery HH, et al. Irs-2 coordinates Igf-1 receptor-mediated beta-cell development and peripheral insulin signalling. Nat Genet 1999;23(1): 32–40.
104. Withers DJ, White MF. Insulin action and type 2 diabetes: lessons from knockout mice. Curr Opin Endocrinol Diabetes 1999;6(2):141–5.
105. Butler RN, Austad SN, Barzilai N, et al. Longevity genes: from primitive organisms to humans. J Gerontol A Biol Sci Med Sci 2003;58(7):581–4.
106. Suh Y, Atzmon G, Cho MO, et al. Functionally significant insulin-like growth factor I receptor mutations in centenarians. Proc Natl Acad Sci U S A 2008; 105(9):3438–42.
107. Willcox BJ, Donlon TA, He Q, et al. FOXO3A genotype is strongly associated with human longevity. Proc Natl Acad Sci U S A 2008;105(37):13987–92.
108. Flachsbart F, Caliebe A, Kleindorp R, et al. Association of FOXO3A variation with human longevity confirmed in German centenarians. Proc Natl Acad Sci U S A 2009;106(8):2700–5.
109. Ling CH, Taekema D, de Craen AJ, et al. Handgrip strength and mortality in the oldest old population: the Leiden 85-plus study. CMAJ 2010;182(5):429–35.
110. Barbieri M, Rizzo MR, Papa M, et al. The IRS2 Gly1057Asp variant is associated with human longevity. J Gerontol A Biol Sci Med Sci 2010;65(3):282–6.
111. Kappeler L, De Magalhaes Filho CM, Dupont J, et al. Brain IGF-1 receptors control mammalian growth and lifespan through a neuroendocrine mechanism. PLoS Biol 2008;6(10):e254.
112. Obici S, Feng Z, Karkanias G, et al. Decreasing hypothalamic insulin receptors causes hyperphagia and insulin resistance in rats. Nat Neurosci 2002;5(6):566–72.
113. Konner AC, Hess S, Tovar S, et al. Role for insulin signaling in catecholaminergic neurons in control of energy homeostasis. Cell Metab 2011;13(6):720–8.
114. Russo SJ, Bolanos CA, Theobald DE, et al. IRS2-Akt pathway in midbrain dopamine neurons regulates behavioral and cellular responses to opiates. Nat Neurosci 2007;10(1):93–9.
115. Choudhury AI, Heffron H, Smith MA, et al. The role of insulin receptor substrate 2 in hypothalamic and beta cell function. J Clin Invest 2005;115(4):940–50.
116. Leininger GM, Myers MG Jr. LRb signals act within a distributed network of leptin-responsive neurones to mediate leptin action. Acta Physiol (Oxf) 2008; 192(1):49–59.
117. Hill JW, Elias CF, Fukuda M, et al. Direct insulin and leptin action on pro-opiomelanocortin neurons is required for normal glucose homeostasis and fertility. Cell Metab 2010;11(4):286–97.
118. Hill JW, Williams KW, Ye C, et al. Acute effects of leptin require PI3K signaling in hypothalamic proopiomelanocortin neurons in mice. J Clin Invest 2008;118(5): 1796–805.
119. Belgardt BF, Husch A, Rother E, et al. PDK1 deficiency in POMC-expressing cells reveals FOXO1-dependent and -independent pathways in control of energy homeostasis and stress response. Cell Metab 2008;7(4):291–301.
120. Al-Qassab H, Smith MA, Irvine EE, et al. Dominant role of the p110beta isoform of PI3K over p110alpha in energy homeostasis regulation by POMC and AgRP neurons. Cell Metab 2009;10(5):343–54.

121. Klockener T, Hess S, Belgardt BF, et al. High-fat feeding promotes obesity via insulin receptor/PI3K-dependent inhibition of SF-1 VMH neurons. Nat Neurosci 2011;14(7):911–8.

122. Myers MG Jr. Leptin receptor signaling and the regulation of mammalian physiology. Recent Prog Horm Res 2004;59:287–304.

123. van de Wall E, Leshan R, Xu AW, et al. Collective and individual functions of leptin receptor modulated neurons controlling metabolism and ingestion. Endocrinology 2008;149(4):1773–85.

124. Bates SH, Myers MG Jr. The role of leptin receptor signaling in feeding and neuroendocrine function. Trends Endocrinol Metab 2003;14(10):447–52.

125. Sadagurski M, Leshan RL, Patterson C, et al. IRS2 signaling in LepR-b neurons suppresses FoxO1 to control energy balance independently of leptin action. Cell Metab 2012;15(5):703–12.

126. Niswender KD, Morton GJ, Stearns WH, et al. Intracellular signalling. Key enzyme in leptin-induced anorexia. Nature 2001;413(6858):794–5.

127. Morton GJ, Gelling RW, Niswender KD, et al. Leptin regulates insulin sensitivity via phosphatidylinositol-3-OH kinase signaling in mediobasal hypothalamic neurons. Cell Metab 2005;2(6):411–20.

128. Dawson TM, Dawson VL. Molecular pathways of neurodegeneration in Parkinson's disease. Science 2003;302(5646):819–22.

129. Selkoe DJ. The molecular pathology of Alzheimer's disease. Neuron 1991;6(4): 487–98.

130. MacDonald ME. Molecular genetics of Huntington's disease. Results Probl Cell Differ 1998;21:47–75.

131. Rozing MP, Westendorp RG, Frolich M, et al. Human insulin/IGF-1 and familial longevity at middle age. Aging (Albany NY) 2009;1(8):714–22.

132. Giannakou ME, Partridge L. Role of insulin-like signalling in *Drosophila* lifespan. Trends Biochem Sci 2007;32(4):180–8.

133. Carro E, Trejo JL, Gomez-Isla T, et al. Serum insulin-like growth factor I regulates brain amyloid-beta levels. Nat Med 2002;8(12):1390–7.

134. Carro E, Trejo JL, Gerber A, et al. Therapeutic actions of insulin-like growth factor I on APP/PS2 mice with severe brain amyloidosis. Neurobiol Aging 2006;27(9):1250–7.

135. Humbert S, Bryson EA, Cordelieres FP, et al. The IGF-1/Akt pathway is neuroprotective in Huntington's disease and involves Huntingtin phosphorylation by Akt. Dev Cell 2002;2(6):831–7.

136. Yamamoto A, Cremona ML, Rothman JE. Autophagy-mediated clearance of huntingtin aggregates triggered by the insulin-signaling pathway. J Cell Biol 2006;172(5):719–31.

137. Amaducci L, Tesco G. Aging as a major risk for degenerative diseases of the central nervous system. Curr Opin Neurol 1994;7(4):283–6.

138. Selkoe DJ. Alzheimer's disease: genes, proteins, and therapy. Physiol Rev 2001; 81(2):741–66.

139. Selkoe DJ. The genetics and molecular pathology of Alzheimer's disease: roles of amyloid and the presenilins. Neurol Clin 2000;18(4):903–22.

140. Pilcher H. Alzheimer's disease could be "type 3 diabetes". Lancet Neurol 2006; 5(5):388–9.

141. Moloney AM, Griffin RJ, Timmons S, et al. Defects in IGF-1 receptor, insulin receptor and IRS-1/2 in Alzheimer's disease indicate possible resistance to IGF-1 and insulin signalling. Neurobiol Aging 2008;31(2):224–43.

142. Copps KD, White MF. Regulation of insulin sensitivity by serine/threonine phosphorylation of insulin receptor substrate proteins IRS1 and IRS2. Diabetologia 2012;55(10):2565–82.
143. Talbot K, Wang HY, Kazi H, et al. Demonstrated brain insulin resistance in Alzheimer's disease patients is associated with IGF-1 resistance, IRS-1 dysregulation, and cognitive decline. J Clin Invest 2012;122(4):1316–38.
144. Bomfim TR, Forny-Germano L, Sathler LB, et al. An anti-diabetes agent protects the mouse brain from defective insulin signaling caused by Alzheimer's disease-associated Abeta oligomers. J Clin Invest 2012;122(4):1339–53.
145. Cohen E, Paulsson JF, Blinder P, et al. Reduced IGF-1 signaling delays age-associated proteotoxicity in mice. Cell 2009;139(6):1157–69.
146. Liu Y, Liu F, Grundke-Iqbal I, et al. Deficient brain insulin signalling pathway in Alzheimer's disease and diabetes. J Pathol 2011;225(1):54–62.
147. Stack EC, Ferrante RJ. Huntington's disease: progress and potential in the field. Expert Opin Investig Drugs 2007;16(12):1933–53.
148. Vonsattel JP, Myers RH, Stevens TJ, et al. Neuropathological classification of Huntington's disease. J Neuropathol Exp Neurol 1985;44(6):559–77.
149. Hockly E, Woodman B, Mahal A, et al. Standardization and statistical approaches to therapeutic trials in the R6/2 mouse. Brain Res Bull 2003;61(5):469–79.
150. Stack EC, Kubilus JK, Smith K, et al. Chronology of behavioral symptoms and neuropathological sequela in R6/2 Huntington's disease transgenic mice. J Comp Neurol 2005;490(4):354–70.
151. Sathasivam K, Lane A, Legleiter J, et al. Identical oligomeric and fibrillar structures captured from the brains of R6/2 and knock-in mouse models of Huntington's disease. Hum Mol Genet 2010;19(1):65–78.
152. St-Pierre J, Drori S, Uldry M, et al. Suppression of reactive oxygen species and neurodegeneration by the PGC-1 transcriptional coactivators. Cell 2006;127(2):397–408.
153. Esposito L, Raber J, Kekonius L, et al. Reduction in mitochondrial superoxide dismutase modulates Alzheimer's disease-like pathology and accelerates the onset of behavioral changes in human amyloid precursor protein transgenic mice. J Neurosci 2006;26(19):5167–79.
154. Gong B, Lim MC, Wanderer J, et al. Time-lapse analysis of aggregate formation in an inducible PC12 cell model of Huntington's disease reveals time-dependent aggregate formation that transiently delays cell death. Brain Res Bull 2008;75(1):146–57.
155. Tabrizi SJ, Workman J, Hart PE, et al. Mitochondrial dysfunction and free radical damage in the Huntington R6/2 transgenic mouse. Ann Neurol 2000;47(1):80–6.
156. Zheng S, Clabough EB, Sarkar S, et al. Deletion of the huntingtin polyglutamine stretch enhances neuronal autophagy and longevity in mice. PLoS Genet 2010;6(2):e1000838.
157. Larsen KE, Sulzer D. Autophagy in neurons: a review. Histol Histopathol 2002;17(3):897–908.
158. Cuervo AM. Autophagy and aging–when "all you can eat" is yourself. Sci Aging Knowledge Environ 2003;2003(36):e25.
159. Mizushima N, Levine B, Cuervo AM, et al. Autophagy fights disease through cellular self-digestion. Nature 2008;451(7182):1069–75.
160. Kang C, You YJ, Avery L. Dual roles of autophagy in the survival of Caenorhabditis elegans during starvation. Genes Dev 2007;21(17):2161–71.

161. Komatsu M, Waguri S, Chiba T, et al. Loss of autophagy in the central nervous system causes neurodegeneration in mice. Nature 2006;441(7095):880–4.
162. Young JE, Martinez RA, La Spada AR. Nutrient deprivation induces neuronal autophagy and implicates reduced insulin signaling in neuroprotective autophagy activation. J Biol Chem 2009;284(4):2363–73.
163. Bjedov I, Toivonen JM, Kerr F, et al. Mechanisms of life span extension by rapamycin in the fruit fly *Drosophila melanogaster*. Cell Metab 2010;11(1):35–46.
164. Di PS, Teutonico A, Leogrande D, et al. Chronic inhibition of mammalian target of rapamycin signaling downregulates insulin receptor substrates 1 and 2 and AKT activation: a crossroad between cancer and diabetes? J Am Soc Nephrol 2006; 17(8):2236–44.
165. Yen WL, Klionsky DJ. How to live long and prosper: autophagy, mitochondria, and aging. Physiology (Bethesda) 2008;23:248–62.
166. Balgi AD, Fonseca BD, Donohue E, et al. Screen for chemical modulators of autophagy reveals novel therapeutic inhibitors of mTORC1 signaling. PLoS One 2009;4(9):e7124.
167. Lamming DW, Ye L, Katajisto P, et al. Rapamycin-induced insulin resistance is mediated by mTORC2 loss and uncoupled from longevity. Science 2012; 335(6076):1638–43.
168. Mojsilovic-Petrovic J, Nedelsky N, Boccitto M, et al. FOXO3a is broadly neuroprotective in vitro and in vivo against insults implicated in motor neuron diseases. J Neurosci 2009;29(25):8236–47.
169. Dillin A, Cohen E. Ageing and protein aggregation-mediated disorders: from invertebrates to mammals. Philos Trans R Soc Lond B Biol Sci 2011; 366(1561):94–8.

Perinatal Programming of Metabolic Diseases

Role of Insulin in the Development of Hypothalamic Neurocircuits

Sophie M. Steculorum, PhD[a,b,c], Merly C. Vogt[a,b,c],
Jens C. Brüning, MD[a,b,c],*

KEYWORDS

- Perinatal programming • Insulin • Glucose • Hypothalamus • Development
- Maternal diabetes • Maternal obesity

KEY POINTS

- Offspring of diabetic mothers are prone to develop metabolic diseases.
- Maternal hyperglycemia leads to compensatory fetal and neonatal hyperinsulinemia.
- Maternal hyperglycemia alters insulin sensing and signaling within the developing hypothalamus.
- Insulin is involved in various steps of hypothalamic development.
- Changes in insulin and/or glucose levels during perinatal life disrupt hypothalamic organization.

INTRODUCTION

It is now generally recognized that obesity and type 2 diabetes mellitus (T2DM) can have their roots even before or just after birth and that alterations of the perinatal environment may predispose to metabolic disorders.[1–4] This perinatal metabolic

Conflict of interest: None.

This work was supported by the Center for Molecular Medicine (CMMC), University of Cologne (TVA1 to J.C.B.), the European Union (FP7/2007-2013 under grant agreement number 241592, EurOCHIP, to J.C.B.), the DFG (BR 1492/7-1 to J.C.B.), and the Competence Network for "Adipositas" (Neurotarget) funded by the Federal Ministry of Education and Research (FKZ01GI0845 to J.C.B.).

[a] Department of Mouse Genetics and Metabolism, Institute for Genetics, Center for Endocrinology, Diabetes and Preventive Medicine (CEDP), University Hospital Cologne and Center for Molecular Medicine Cologne (CMMC), University of Cologne, Zülpicher Street 47a, Köln 50674, Germany; [b] Cologne Excellence Cluster on Cellular Stress Responses in Aging Associated Diseases (CECAD), Zülpicher Street 47a, Köln 50674, Germany; [c] Max-Planck-Institute for Neurological Research, Gleueler Street 50a, Köln 50931, Germany

* Corresponding author. Max-Planck-Institute for Neurologic Research, Gleueler Street 50a, Köln 50931, Germany.

E-mail address: bruening@nf.mpg.de

Endocrinol Metab Clin N Am 42 (2013) 149–164
http://dx.doi.org/10.1016/j.ecl.2012.10.002
0889-8529/13/$ – see front matter © 2013 Elsevier Inc. All rights reserved.

programming significantly contributes to the dramatic increase in the incidences of obesity and its associated diseases observed across the past decades. Predictive studies estimate that if the increasing trend of obesity prevalence continues, more than half of the American adults will be obese by 2030.[5] Obesity and T2DM occur consistently earlier in life and have also reached an alarming prevalence in children and teenagers.[6–9] Childhood obesity and/or glucose intolerance have been shown to be valuable predictors of the onset of metabolic diseases in adults.[10–12] The Bogalusa study revealed that the risk of developing metabolic diseases is 8 times increased in adults with a history of overweight during childhood.[10] The notion that perinatal programming substantially contributes to the cause of obesity has lead to a multitude of clinical, epidemiologic, and animal studies aiming to better define the molecular mechanisms underlying the programming of metabolic diseases.

EVIDENCE OF PERINATAL ORIGINS OF METABOLIC DISEASES
Historical Background

As early as the sixties, Dubos and colleagues[13] indicated that changes in maternal nutritional status during gestation and/or lactation in rodents could affect lifelong body weight regulation of the offspring. Despite several other studies highlighting a link between early life events and later diseases, Barker and Hales pioneered the concept of perinatal programming. Based on epidemiologic data, they demonstrated that low-birth-weight babies (ie, born form malnourished mothers) have an increased risk of developing cardiovascular diseases, diabetes, and obesity.[14–16] This correlation between low birth weight and metabolic outcomes led to the so-called Barker hypothesis, which postulated that development in a poor environment leads to developmental adaptive responses that optimize growth and survival; however, when exposed to more abundant nutrition later in life, these adaptations become detrimental and induce metabolic diseases.[17]

General Concept of Perinatal Programming

The concept of metabolic imprinting by the perinatal environment has been expanded to several nutritional and hormonal insults including maternal obesity and diabetes. Numerous studies demonstrate that offspring of mothers with obesity and/or diabetes (type 1, type 2, and gestational diabetes) are prone to develop metabolic disorders later in life.[18–23] The relationship between birth weight/maternal nutritional status and adult risk to develop metabolic diseases can be summarized by a U-shaped curve: the susceptibility toward developing obesity and/or T2DM is increased for both low-birth-weight and macrosomic babies from undernourished and overnourished mothers, respectively. Similarly, hypoinsulinemia and hyperinsulinemia during development may cause metabolic diseases later in life. This predisposing effect of perinatal environment on the metabolic fate of the offspring presumably reflects interference with fundamental developmental processes. Furthermore, it emphasizes the developmental plasticity of each organism by demonstrating that a given genotype has the ability to give rise to more than 1 phenotype depending on the environmental milieu.[24] Among all the organs playing a key role in the regulation of metabolic functions, particular attention has been paid to the developmental programming of the hypothalamic network controlling appetite and glucose homeostasis.

HYPOTHALAMIC REGULATION OF ENERGY BALANCE AND GLUCOSE HOMEOSTASIS

Central control of energy balance and glucose homeostasis involves highly complex mechanisms that are beyond the scope of this review but that have been extensively reviewed elsewhere.[25–28] In a simplistic view, the hypothalamic control of appetite and glycemia is mediated by a range of neuropeptides expressed in several key hypothalamic nuclei such as the arcuate nucleus (ARH), the lateral hypothalamic area (LHA), and the dorsomedial (DMH), the ventromedial (VMH), and the paraventricular (PVH) nuclei of the hypothalamus. Because of the close proximity of the ARH to the median eminence and its permeable microvasculature, it is the primary target of blood-borne signals.[29] The ARH contains 2 main functionally antagonistic neuronal populations: the orexigenic neurons coexpressing neuropeptide Y (NPY) and agouti-related peptide (AgRP) and the anorexigenic neurons that produce pro-opiomelanocortin (POMC) and cocaine and amphetamine regulated transcript (CART). These 2 populations of neurons are direct targets of the adipocyte-derived hormone leptin and the pancreatic hormone insulin. Leptin and insulin stimulate POMC neurons, whereas they inhibit NPY/AgRP neurons to mediate their anorexigenic effect and to increase energy expenditure. POMC and NPY/AgRP neurons send intensive and convergent projections to other hypothalamic nuclei, notably to the DMH, PVH, and LHA. More specifically, these projections target other key neurons containing orexigenic peptides, such as the melanin-concentrating hormone (MCH) and the orexins in the LHA, and anorexigenic peptides including thyrotropin-releasing hormone (TRH) and corticotropin-releasing hormone (CRH) located in the PVH. Activation or inhibition of these neurons (either by arcuate neuronal projections or by a direct action of peripheral hormones) results in endocrine, autonomic, and behavioral responses leading to the regulation of energy balance and glucose homeostasis.[25–28]

DEVELOPMENT OF HYPOTHALAMIC FEEDING NETWORK IN RODENTS

Hypothalamic development follows 2 major steps: first, the determination of neuronal cell number that includes neurogenesis, neuronal differentiation, and migration, and second, the formation of functional networks with the ontogeny of neuronal projections and formation of synapses (**Fig. 1**). These 2 steps are common in all species; however, the developmental time frame differs depending on the species: in humans and nonhuman primates the hypothalamus is relatively mature at birth, whereas development of the hypothalamus occurs both during gestation and lactation in rodents.[30–32] As most of the animal models of perinatal programming are established in mice or rats, hypothalamic development in rodents is described in further detail in the following section. Nonetheless, species consideration and human data are discussed later.

Ontogeny of Hypothalamic Neurons

The mediobasal hypothalamus develops from the diencephalic vesicle, which is formed around embryonic day 12 (E12) in rodents.[33–35] Hypothalamic neurons originate from the proliferative zone of the neuroepithelium of the third ventricle and then migrate to their target area (see **Fig. 1**).[33–36] Formation of hypothalamic neurons follows an "outside-in" pattern, with the more lateral structures forming before the more medial.[33–37] Neurogenesis in rodents occurs between E12 and E16/E17, with a peak of neuron formation at E12 (see **Fig. 1**). In line with the lateromedial gradient of neurogenesis, neurons located in the LHA are born at E12 with a short neurogenic period. Neurons that form the PVH and the DMH form between E12 and E16. The last wave of neurogenesis occurs between E12 and E16/E17 and is devoted to neurons that take residence in the more medial region (ie, ARH and VMH).[33–37]

Cell fate of hypothalamic neurons seems to be determined early after neurogenesis, as several neuropeptides (including MCH, TRH, and CRH) have been detected in

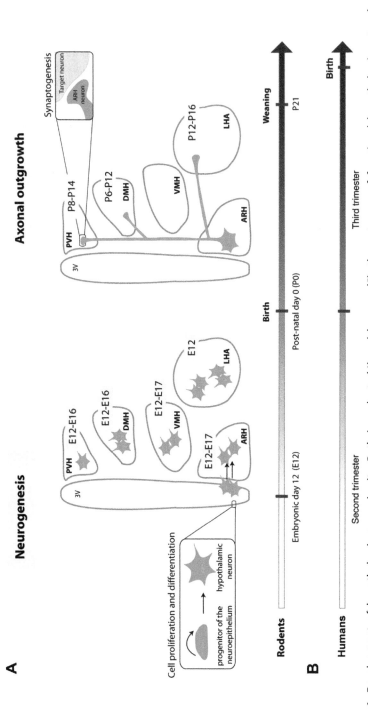

Fig. 1. Development of hypothalamic neurocircuits. Both in rodents (*A*) and humans (*B*), the ontogeny of functional hypothalamic networks is composed of 2 major steps: (1) the birth of neurons (ie, neurogenesis) directly followed by their differentiation and migration and (2) the formation of mature axonal projections that include axonal outgrowth and synaptogenesis. In rodents (*A*), hypothalamic neurons originate from progenitor cells of the neuroepithelium of the third ventricle that are generated between embryonic day 12 (E12) and E17 depending on the area. In rodents, development of axonal projections from arcuate neurons occurs during the first weeks of life; once arcuate projections reach their target neurons they develop synaptic contact. Hypothalamic development occurs both during gestation and lactation in rodents and is not mature before weaning, whereas in humans (*B*), the hypothalamus is mature at birth as neurogenesis and axonal outgrowth, respectively, take place during the second and the third trimesters. E, embryonic day; P, postnatal day; 3V, third ventricle.

neurons right after their formation.[38–40] Padilla and colleagues[36] demonstrated that NPY and POMC neurons display a specific profile of differentiation, with nearly one-quarter of mature NPY neurons sharing a common progenitor with POMC cells.

Ontogeny of Functional Neuronal Network

In rodents, the formation of hypothalamic neural projections occurs during fetal and neonatal life depending on the specific networks, resulting in the establishment of a fully mature core circuitry by the third week of postnatal life.

Neural projections from the ARH develop during neonatal life when at postnatal day 4 (P4) arcuate neurons start to emit projections through the periventricular zone of the third ventricle to successively reach the DMH at P6, the PVH at P8, and finally the LHA at P12; ARH projections to these area are, respectively, mature by P12, P14, and P16 (see **Fig. 1**).[30] Neuronal projections from the ARH fully develop and acquire an adultlike profile by P18.[30] There is a paucity of data regarding the exact timing of the formation of VMH and DMH projections; however, axonal labeling experiments showed that projections from these nuclei to the PVH are fully mature by P6 and P10, respectively.[30] Intrahypothalamic projections seem to develop mainly after birth, whereas efferent and afferent inputs between the brain stem and the PVH are formed during fetal life and are fully mature at birth.[41] Accordingly, infusions of NPY to the PVH in neonates induce an increase in food intake,[42] showing that PVH downstream networks controlling appetite are fully mature at birth. In contrast, leptin has no anorexigenic effect before ARH projections acquire a mature pattern, suggesting that the development of ARH projections represents a key step and seems essential for the integration of hormonal peripheral signals.[43] Synaptogenesis in the mediobasal hypothalamus is poorly described but seems to occur late, as, for instance, only half of the synapses in the ARH are detectable at weaning, whereas they are fully developed by P45.[44,45]

In summary, hypothalamic development occurs during 2 different periods of life in rodents and is therefore exposed to 2 successive environments that represent critical periods of vulnerability. Wiring of hypothalamic networks is governed by a range of molecules including hormonal factors. In the context of perinatal programming, particular attention has been paid to hormones that not only are sensitive to pathologic and nutritional status but also exert some developmental actions. Leptin and insulin are known to play a dual role on hypothalamic circuits: in addition to acting on the mature hypothalamic network to regulate feeding and glucose metabolism in the adult organism, leptin and insulin also act within the developing hypothalamus to govern its development. The neurodevelopmental actions of leptin have been extensively reviewed elsewhere (see Refs.[46,47]); therefore, this review particularly focuses on the role of insulin in the development of hypothalamic circuits and on the structural and functional consequences of maternal diabetes on these networks. As particular attention is paid on the consequences of perinatal hyperinsulinemia secondary to maternal hyperglycemia, type 1 and type 2 maternal diabetes are simultaneously discussed in this review; nonetheless, known differences between maternal hypoinsulinemia and hyperinsulinemia are stated.

IMPORTANCE OF PERINATAL INSULIN AND GLUCOSE LEVELS IN THE PROGRAMMING OF HYPOTHALAMIC CIRCUITS IN RODENTS
Influence of Perinatal Environment on Fetal and Neonatal Insulin Levels

The ability to secrete insulin is acquired early during fetal development both in humans and in rodents.[48,49] Although the pancreatic insulin secretory machinery is not fully matured during fetal and neonatal life in rodents, insulin secretion already depends on increasing circulating glucose levels.[50] Moreover, maternal insulin cannot cross the placental barrier, whereas maternal glucose is actively transported to the fetus, where it acts to stimulate insulin secretion.[51,52] Consistently, maternal hyperglycemia results in compensatory fetal hyperinsulinemia. This adaptive endocrine response sets the basis for the Pedersen hypothesis that fetal hyperinsulinemia is the main factor responsible for the detrimental effects on the metabolic phenotypes observed in offspring of diabetic mothers.[53,54] Mild hyperglycemia induced by glucose infusion during the last week of gestation in rats is sufficient to induce neonatal hyperinsulinemia and long-term impairment of glucose homeostasis in the offspring.[55] Particularly troublesome, fetal hyperinsulinemia occurs not only under chronic maternal hyperglycemia but also in response to short-term increases in glucose levels. Leloup and colleagues[56] used a hyperglycemic clamp during the last 48 hours of gestation and demonstrated that fetal insulin concentrations are increased nearly 7-fold in response to transient mild maternal hyperglycemia in rats.

The Pedersen hypothesis, as well as the critical role of maternal glucose levels during the offspring's development, demonstrates the necessity for well-balanced maternal insulin levels during pregnancy. Various studies performed in rodents demonstrated that maternal insulin deficiency and insulin resistance result in maternal hyperglycemia and subsequently induce fetal and neonatal hyperinsulinemia, a condition that has been shown to predispose the offspring for obesity and diabetes.[57-61] Increased insulin levels are also detected within the hypothalamus of newborn pups of diabetic mothers, showing that hypothalamic development is directly targeted by this hyperinsulinemia.[57]

Insulin Signaling Within the Developing Hypothalamus

Insulin receptors (IRs) are highly expressed within the developing brain including the hypothalamus.[62,63] In rodents, expression levels of brain IRs reach a maximum during the last week of gestation and then decrease to adult levels during the first days of life.[63] Accordingly, binding of insulin to its receptors follows a similar pattern,[64] which is likely due to the increased expression of IRs because the affinity of the receptors remains constant throughout life.[64] In addition to the developmental upregulation of the IRs, access and binding of insulin to its receptors in the developing brain seem to be further facilitated by the immaturity of the blood–brain barrier.[65]

The functionality of IRs in fetal and neonatal brains has been demonstrated by the ability of insulin to autophosphorylate the IR β-subunits.[64] Moreover, the presence of competent IRs within the hypothalamus has also been highlighted by the ability of fetal intracerebroventricular administration of insulin to reduce NPY levels.[66] This developmental upregulation of insulin sensing and signaling before birth is specific to the brain, as IR autophosphorylation remains constant throughout development in other classic insulin-sensitive organs such as the liver.[64]

Development under abnormally high nutrient and hormone levels leads to immediate alterations of insulin sensing and actions. Fetal hyperinsulinemia is accompanied by an increased insulin concentration within the developing hypothalamus. Furthermore, maternal hyperglycemia increases insulin binding in various hypothalamic nuclei including the ARH (**Fig. 2**).[56] Accordingly, expression of hypothalamic IRs is elevated in term fetuses of hyperinsulinemic mothers.[59] The same study, as well as others conducted in preweaning pups of mothers with obesity, demonstrates that despite the increased expression of IRs, the levels of the downstream signaling molecules, insulin receptors substrate 2 and mammalian target of rapamycin are decreased, suggesting that maternal obesity may affect insulin signaling and lead to

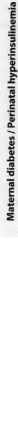
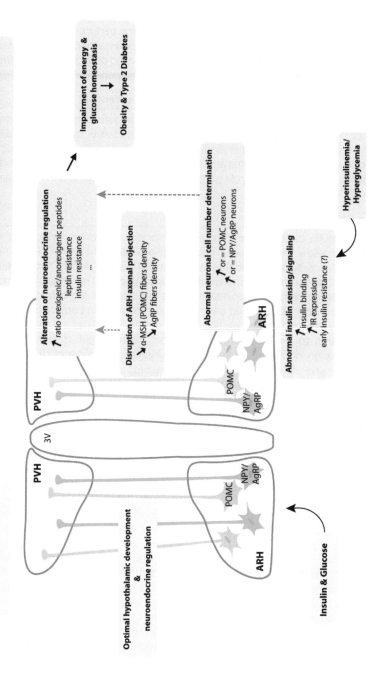

Fig. 2. Structural and functional consequences of maternal diabetes on hypothalamic neurocircuits controlling energy and glucose homeostasis. Perinatal hyperinsulinemia, secondary to maternal diabetes, leads to abnormal insulin sensing and signaling during critical periods of hypothalamic development. Architectural alterations of hypothalamic neurocircuits, including abnormal neuronal cell number determination and disruption of axonal projections from arcuate neurons, have been described in different rodent models of maternal diabetes. These neurodevelopmental defects may contribute to various alterations of neuroendocrine regulation reported in offspring of diabetic mothers and therefore to the onset of obesity and type 2 diabetes. For corresponding references, please see the main text. 3V, third ventricle; α-MSH, α-melanocyte-stimulating hormone.

an early hypothalamic insulin resistance.[59,61,67] However, due to the paucity of data regarding the effect of maternal diabetes on perinatal insulin sensitivity, it is challenging to draw further conclusions, and additional studies are required to address this question.

In summary, exposure to a diabetogenic environment perturbs perinatal insulin secretion, giving rise to peripheral and hypothalamic hyperinsulinemia and to premature disruptions of hypothalamic insulin sensing and signaling during critical periods of neuronal circuitry ontogeny.

Neurodevelopmental Actions of Insulin on Hypothalamic Network

Basic knowledge regarding the involvement of insulin on hypothalamic development is surprisingly poor, and only few studies, mainly performed in vitro, describe the role of insulin on the ontogeny of hypothalamic networks. However, experiments conducted in rodent models of maternal diabetes and/or perinatal hyperinsulinemia provide valuable information regarding the key role of insulin on the various steps of hypothalamic development.

Cell Number Determination

Both maternal insulin deficiency and insulin resistance have been associated with changes in hypothalamic neuronal cell number. In this context, the work of Plagemann and colleagues has provided a substantial amount of data regarding hypothalamic "malorganization" secondary to maternal hypoinsulinemia. The most commonly used animal model of maternal hypoinsulinemia is induced by injections of the beta-cell toxin streptozotocin (STZ) during early gestation resulting in beta-cell death and subsequent hyperglycemia. However, application of this model has led to conflicting results with regards to its effect on hypothalamic neuronal cell number. On one hand, STZ application in pregnant dams led to an increased number of NPY neurons within the ARH of juvenile offspring of diabetic mothers;[57] on the other hand, it was reported to result in an elevated number of POMC but not NPY neurons, which was further supported by a genetic model of maternal insulin resistance (see **Fig. 2**).[68,69] These discrepancies presumably originate from species differences (rats vs mice) and/or from the intensity of the maternal diabetes (mild vs severe). Although these studies clearly demonstrate that maternal diabetes alters the determination of hypothalamic neuronal number, they do not address the exact origin of the observed changes. The work of Desai and colleagues[70] revealed that insulin promotes neurogenesis on fetal hypothalamic progenitor neurospheres, strongly suggesting that changes in hypothalamic neuronal number can be attributed, at least in part, to changes in neurogenesis. Plum and colleagues[71] used genetic approaches to invalidate hypothalamic IRs and mimic their constitutive activation in POMC neurons and found that loss and gain of function of IRs led to an increase and a decrease of arcuate POMC cell number, respectively. However, in this study, these differences were not detectable during development but only during adult life, suggesting that insulin is involved in the regulation of neuronal pool size in adult rather than in fetal neurogenesis. Thus, further investigation is needed to decipher the role of insulin signaling during development in determining neuronal cell number of hypothalamic neurocircuits. Moreover, maternal diabetes also alters hypothalamic catecholaminergic systems as revealed by an increased number of tyrosine hydroxylase-containing neurons in the arcuate and periventricular nuclei and by abnormal levels of norepinephrine and dopamine in various hypothalamic regions.[58,72,73] Particular attention has also been paid to the VMH, as it is well known to be involved in the central action of insulin. VMH of offspring of diabetic mothers show several neuroanatomic aberrations including a decreased number of neurons.[58,74,75] In addition to modulating the number of neurons per se, maternal diabetes also induces more profound changes on the overall morphology of hypothalamic nuclei and on the neuronal cytoarchitecture such as neuronal dysplasia and hypotrophy.[58,74,75] Normalization of maternal glucose levels by pancreatic islet transplantation during the second week of gestation prevents the hypothalamic malorganization described earlier, emphasizing the key programming effect of maternal glucose and/or fetal insulin levels in hypothalamic development.[74–76]

Hypothalamic neuronal number is further affected when offspring are exposed to a diabetic environment exclusively during lactation. When raised by diabetic mothers, weanling rats born from control mothers display decreased POMC and increased galanin neurons within the ARH.[77] This study suggests that a diabetogenic environment may also change the neuronal pool number in a manner different from its effects on neurogenesis, possibly by modulating neonatal neuronal death and/or survival.

Neuronal Circuits Formation

Insulin is known to act as a neurotrophic factor during brain development, including that of the developing hypothalamus. In vitro experiments revealed that insulin promotes neurite elongation of hypothalamic neurons (both fetal neurons and organotypic explants).[78,79] Elevation of neonatal insulin levels by subcutaneous injections of insulin during the critical period of axonal projection formation induces long-term metabolic outcomes such as obesity or glucose intolerance.[80] Hyperinsulinemia specifically and exclusively within the mediobasal hypothalamus for a period of 4 days is sufficient to recapitulate all the metabolic outcomes and the neurodevelopmental alterations observed in offspring of diabetic mothers.[81,82] These data strongly suggest that the abnormal action of insulin on hypothalamic neurons is largely responsible for the perinatal programming of metabolism. In addition, disruption of hypothalamic circuit organization has been reported in rodent models of maternal hypoinsulinemia and hyperinsulinemia.[69,83,84] In both cases, the fiber density of arcuate POMC and NPY/AgRP neurons innervating the paraventricular nucleus was reduced in offspring of diabetic mothers (see **Fig. 2**).[69,83,84] Despite an increase in the number of arcuate POMC neurons, offspring of hypoinsulinemic mothers display a decrease in α-melanocyte-stimulating hormone fiber density, suggesting that the reduction of fiber density may be due to a defect of axonal outgrowth rather than a reduced number of neurons.[69]

Altogether, data obtained from different models of maternal diabetes clearly show that exposure to hyperglycemia and/or hyperinsulinemia during perinatal development permanently affects the organization of hypothalamic networks (see **Fig. 2**), suggesting a key role for glucose and insulin in this neurodevelopmental programming. In addition to insulin, a large range of hormonal factors acts antagonistically and synergistically to shape neuronal networks (for review see Refs.[85,86]). Considering that maternal hyperglycemia is accompanied by a multitude of endocrine and metabolic changes, including a variation of leptinemia and lipid profiles, many other factors may also contribute to the full manifestation of these "malprogramming" processes. In both models of maternal diabetes (hypoinsulinemia and hyperinsulinemia), leptin resistance has been reported in the ARH of neonates.[69,83,84] In contrast to type 1 diabetes, T2DM commonly occurs secondary to increased weight gain and adiposity, and it is thereby associated with a widespread metabolic signature that includes lipid excess and upregulation of adipocyte-secreted factors.[87] Therefore, additional studies are required to address the exact programming effect of maternal obesity per se, independent of diabetes, as well as the distinct role of insulin on hypothalamic development and its interaction with other developmental factors.

MECHANISTIC ASPECTS OF HYPOTHALAMIC PROGRAMMING

Mechanisms underlying the programming of neuroendocrine hypothalamic networks are poorly understood. Strikingly, the major hallmarks of obesity and T2DM in adults have been reported during development in various animal models of programming. Exposure to perinatal hyperglycemia and/or hyperinsulinemia led to premature and permanent impairments of neuroendocrine hypothalamic functions that are presumably involved in the onset of obesity and glucose intolerance. As described previously, secondary to maternal diabetes, perinatal levels of insulin are elevated and insulin signaling within the fetal hypothalamus seems to be altered. Electrophysiological recordings performed in a model of neonatal overnutrition revealed that hyperinsulinemia is associated with premature insulin resistance of arcuate neurons that persists throughout adulthood.[88] Accordingly, an imbalance in the expression of appetite-regulatory neuropeptides has been reported in the hypothalami of hyperinsulinemic fetuses and juvenile rats, resulting in a greater ratio of orexigenic to anorexigenic peptide expression (see **Fig. 2**).[59,61,67,89] Finally, another striking example of the "obesogenic profile" of programmed hypothalami is the upregulation of several inflammatory pathways in the hypothalami of offspring from mothers fed a high-fat diet (HFD).[90] In this study, Rother and colleagues[90] reported an increased activation of the inflammation-mediated kinases c-Jun N-terminal kinase1 and Iκ-kinase-β under basal condition in offspring from HFD-fed mothers, highlighting that maternal overnutrition leads to a constitutive hypothalamic inflammation in the offspring. Accordingly, upregulation of proinflammatory markers has also been described in hypothalami of nonhuman primate fetuses of HFD-fed mothers with obesity.[91] Cellular inflammation could also be triggered by the increased number of reactive oxygen species (ROS) in response to hyperglycemia (for review see Refs.[92,93]). Although basal levels of oxidative stress are required for an optimal organogenesis, abnormally elevated redox states compromise embryonic development.[92,93] For instance, exposure to excessive levels of oxidative stress during fetal life alters the development and thus function of pancreatic beta-cells.[92,93] Despite data showing that physiologic levels of ROS play a regulatory role in the development of the central nervous system (including in neurogenesis and cell fate), the consequences of aberrant ROS signaling and mitochondrial dysfunctions in the malprogramming of hypothalamic circuits have not been investigated.[92–94]

CRITICAL PERIOD OF HYPOTHALAMIC DEVELOPMENT: SPECIES CONSIDERATIONS

While hypothalamic development takes place between gestational and neonatal stages in rodents, it is restricted to in utero life in humans and nonhuman primates (see **Fig. 1**).[31,95] In all species, neuronal birth occurs during fetal life; however, marked developmental divergence lies in the timing of axonal projection formation.[30,31,95] Both in humans and nonhuman primates, neurogenesis of hypothalamic neurons occurs during the middle of the second trimester directly followed by the development of their axonal projections that continues throughout the third trimester (see **Fig. 1**).[31,32,95] Although arcuate projections are nearly mature at birth in nonhuman primates, they pursue their development during neonatal life, suggesting that early life is also critical for the maturation of hypothalamic networks in higher species.[31] Accordingly, it is recognized that both gestation and early infancy represent critical periods of sensitivity for the later onset of obesity in humans.

For obvious ethical concerns, the effect of hormonal and nutritional environment on hypothalamic neurocircuit development has never been assessed in humans. However, data provided in nonhuman primates reported identical neurodevelopmental alterations to the ones described in rodents.[91] For instance, Grayson and colleagues[91] demonstrated that arcuate projections are decreased in nonhuman primate fetuses of mothers with obesity. Naturally, these data do not warrant that similar events occur in humans but emphasize that malprogramming of the hypothalamus in response to an abnormal nutritional environment also happens in nonhuman primates that share common timing of hypothalamic development with humans.

CONCLUSIONS AND FUTURE PERSPECTIVES

In summary, it is clear from human and animal studies that the perinatal hormonal environment is critical for the metabolic fate of an individual. Increased perinatal glucose levels secondary to maternal diabetes lead to abnormal wiring of hypothalamic feeding circuits. This pivotal role of the maternal glycemic index explains how a surfeit and a paucity of maternal insulin can lead to similar neurodevelopmental and pathologic outcomes. Compensatory perinatal hyperinsulinemia seems to be largely responsible for the structural and functional abnormalities as observed in cases of maternal hyperglycemia, highlighting the key regulatory role of insulin on various steps of hypothalamic ontogeny including neurogenesis and axonal outgrowth.

Although developmental processes underlying this metabolic imprinting are far from being completely understood, it is clear that diabetes during pregnancy leads to a greater susceptibility to detrimental metabolic outcomes in the offspring, including in humans. Increasingly more women in childbearing age are obese and/or diabetic, suggesting that their children will likely develop metabolic diseases that will obviously contribute to the estimated increase in the prevalence of obesity expected in the coming years. Thus, one of the key questions that need to be assessed is, How to prevent this perinatal imprinting? One big step toward prevention could be via specific nutritional intervention during pregnancy, as it has been shown to reverse the predisposition of offspring from overnourished mothers with obesity in nonhuman primates.[91] Remarkably, healthy nutrient consumption exclusively during pregnancy is able to rescue the developmental hypothalamic alterations in nonhuman primate fetuses of mothers with obesity, including a normalization of the hypothalamic circuit's organization.[91] In contrast, HFD consumption exclusively during gestation in lean rats has dramatic effects on hypothalamic neurocircuit development and lifelong metabolism.[96] In an optimistic view, these results raise the promise that malprogramming events may be preventable by dietary management before or during pregnancy. However, they also highlight the extreme sensitivity of hypothalamic ontogeny to nutritional and hormonal developmental milieu. As described previously, perturbation of neuronal development does not only occur secondary to chronic environmental alterations but can also be induced by acute and/or episodic changes in perinatal hormonal status. This situation is of a particular concern for offspring of insulin-treated mothers that experience mild exposure to hyperglycemia or hypoglycemia. Although efforts are put into the prevention of maternal hyperglycemia, hypoglycemia also has a teratogenic effect on fetal development (for review see Refs.[97,98]). Thus, strict prevention of dietary and hormonal variations in humans does not seem as trivial considering the difficulties to tightly control glycemia under diabetic conditions, as well as the social and hedonic regulation of appetite. Therefore, it is of great importance to better define the exact molecular mechanisms underlying the programming of metabolic neuronal networks including hormonal mediators, their intracellular signaling, and the precise neurodevelopmental outputs. Ultimately, deciphering the exact mechanisms responsible for these malprogramming events may not only lead to new potential therapeutic approaches but may also advance the basic knowledge regarding fundamental key aspects of brain development.

ACKNOWLEDGMENTS

The authors apologize to those colleagues whose important contributions could not be cited because of space limitations. They thank Gisela Schmall and Tanja Rayle for excellent secretarial assistance.

REFERENCES

1. McMillen IC, Robinson JS. Developmental origins of the metabolic syndrome: prediction, plasticity, and programming. Physiol Rev 2005;85(2):571–633.
2. Plagemann A. Perinatal nutrition and hormone-dependent programming of food intake. Horm Res 2006;65(Suppl 3):83–9.
3. Levin BE. Metabolic imprinting: critical impact of the perinatal environment on the regulation of energy homeostasis. Philos Trans R Soc Lond B Biol Sci 2006; 361(1471):1107–21.
4. Fernandez-Twinn DS, Ozanne SE. Early life nutrition and metabolic programming. Ann N Y Acad Sci 2010;1212:78–96.
5. Wang Y, Beydoun MA, Liang L, et al. Will all Americans become overweight or obese? Estimating the progression and cost of the US obesity epidemic. Obesity (Silver Spring) 2008;16(10):2323–30.
6. Ebbeling CB, Pawlak DB, Ludwig DS. Childhood obesity: public-health crisis, common sense cure. Lancet 2002;360(9331):473–82.
7. Ludwig DS, Ebbeling CB. Type 2 diabetes mellitus in children: primary care and public health considerations. JAMA 2001;286(12):1427–30.
8. Hedley AA, Ogden CL, Johnson CL, et al. Prevalence of overweight and obesity among US children, adolescents, and adults, 1999-2002. JAMA 2004;291(23):2847–50.
9. Sabin MA, Shield JP. Childhood obesity. Front Horm Res 2008;36:85–96.
10. Srinivasan SR, Bao W, Wattigney WA, et al. Adolescent overweight is associated with adult overweight and related multiple cardiovascular risk factors: the Bogalusa Heart Study. Metabolism 1996;45(2):235–40.
11. Whitaker RC, Wright JA, Pepe MS, et al. Predicting obesity in young adulthood from childhood and parental obesity. N Engl J Med 1997;337(13):869–73.
12. Berenson GS, Radhakrishnamurthy B, Bao W, et al. Does adult-onset diabetes mellitus begin in childhood? The Bogalusa Heart Study. Am J Med Sci 1995; 310(Suppl 1):S77–82.
13. Dubos R, Savage D, Schaedler R. Biological Freudianism. Lasting effects of early environmental influences. Pediatrics 1966;38(5):789–800.
14. Barker DJ, Osmond C, Golding J, et al. Growth in utero, blood pressure in childhood and adult life, and mortality from cardiovascular disease. BMJ 1989; 298(6673):564–7.
15. Osmond C, Barker DJ, Slattery JM. Risk of death from cardiovascular disease and chronic bronchitis determined by place of birth in England and Wales. J Epidemiol Community Health 1990;44(2):139–41.
16. Hales CN, Barker DJ, Clark PM, et al. Fetal and infant growth and impaired glucose tolerance at age 64. BMJ 1991;303(6809):1019–22.
17. Hales CN, Barker DJ. Type 2 (non-insulin-dependent) diabetes mellitus: the thrifty phenotype hypothesis. Diabetologia 1992;35(7):595–601.
18. Berenson GS, Bao W, Srinivasan SR. Abnormal characteristics in young offspring of parents with non-insulin-dependent diabetes mellitus. The Bogalusa Heart Study. Am J Epidemiol 1996;144(10):962–7.
19. Jovanovic L, Pettitt DJ. Gestational diabetes mellitus. JAMA 2001;286(20): 2516–8.

20. Plagemann A, Harder T, Kohlhoff R, et al. Overweight and obesity in infants of mothers with long-term insulin-dependent diabetes or gestational diabetes. Int J Obes Relat Metab Disord 1997;21(6):451–6.
21. Pedersen JF. Ultrasound studies on fetal crown-rump length in early normal and diabetic pregnancy. Dan Med Bull 1986;33(6):296–304.
22. Boney CM, Verma A, Tucker R, et al. Metabolic syndrome in childhood: association with birth weight, maternal obesity, and gestational diabetes mellitus. Pediatrics 2005;115(3):e290–6.
23. Gibson LY, Byrne SM, Davis EA, et al. The role of family and maternal factors in childhood obesity. Med J Aust 2007;186(11):591–5.
24. Barker DJ. Developmental origins of adult health and disease. J Epidemiol Community Health 2004;58(2):114–5.
25. Berthoud HR. Multiple neural systems controlling food intake and body weight. Neurosci Biobehav Rev 2002;26(4):393–428.
26. Elmquist JK, Elias CF, Saper CB. From lesions to leptin: hypothalamic control of food intake and body weight. Neuron 1999;22(2):221–32.
27. Konner AC, Klockener T, Bruning JC. Control of energy homeostasis by insulin and leptin: targeting the arcuate nucleus and beyond. Physiol Behav 2009; 97(5):632–8.
28. Elmquist JK, Coppari R, Balthasar N, et al. Identifying hypothalamic pathways controlling food intake, body weight, and glucose homeostasis. J Comp Neurol 2005;493(1):63–71.
29. Ciofi P, Garret M, Lapirot O, et al. Brain-endocrine interactions: a microvascular route in the mediobasal hypothalamus. Endocrinology 2009;150(12):5509–19.
30. Bouret SG, Draper SJ, Simerly RB. Formation of projection pathways from the arcuate nucleus of the hypothalamus to hypothalamic regions implicated in the neural control of feeding behavior in mice. J Neurosci 2004;24(11):2797–805.
31. Grayson BE, Allen SE, Billes SK, et al. Prenatal development of hypothalamic neuropeptide systems in the nonhuman primate. Neuroscience 2006;143(4): 975–86.
32. Koutcherov Y, Mai JK, Paxinos G. Hypothalamus of the human fetus. J Chem Neuroanat 2003;26(4):253–70.
33. Altman J, Bayer S. The development of the rat hypothalamus. Adv Anat Embryol Cell Biol 1986;100(100):178.
34. Ifft JD. An autoradiographic study of the time of final division of neurons in rat hypothalamic nuclei. J Comp Neurol 1972;144(2):193–204.
35. Shimada M, Nakamura T. Time of neuron origin in mouse hypothalamic nuclei. Exp Neurol 1973;41(1):163–73.
36. Padilla SL, Carmody JS, Zeltser LM. POMC-expressing progenitors give rise to antagonistic neuronal populations in hypothalamic feeding circuits. Nat Med 2010;16(4):403–5.
37. Ishii Y, Bouret SG. Embryonic birthdate of hypothalamic leptin-activated neurons in mice. Endocrinology 2012;153:3657–67.
38. Brischoux F, Fellmann D, Risold PY. Ontogenetic development of the diencephalic MCH neurons: a hypothalamic 'MCH area' hypothesis. Eur J Neurosci 2001;13(9):1733–44.
39. Burgunder JM, Taylor T. Ontogeny of thyrotropin-releasing hormone gene expression in the rat diencephalon. Neuroendocrinology 1989;49(6):631–40.
40. Daikoku S, Okamura Y, Kawano H, et al. Immunohistochemical study on the development of CRF-containing neurons in the hypothalamus of the rat. Cell Tissue Res 1984;238(3):539–44.

41. Lakke EA, Hinderink JB. Development of the spinal projections of the nucleus paraventricularis hypothalami of the rat: an intra-uterine WGA-HRP study. Brain Res Dev Brain Res 1989;49(1):115–21.

42. Capuano CA, Leibowitz SF, Barr GA. Effect of paraventricular injection of neuropeptide Y on milk and water intake of preweanling rats. Neuropeptides 1993;24(3):177–82.

43. Ahima RS, Prabakaran D, Flier JS. Postnatal leptin surge and regulation of circadian rhythm of leptin by feeding. Implications for energy homeostasis and neuroendocrine function. J Clin Invest 1998;101(5):1020–7.

44. Koritsanszky S. Cyto- and synaptogenesis in the arcuate nucleus of the rat hypothalamus during fetal and early postnatal life. Cell Tissue Res 1979;200(1):135–46.

45. Matsumoto A, Arai Y. Developmental changes in synaptic formation in the hypothalamic arcuate nucleus of female rats. Cell Tissue Res 1976;169(2):143–56.

46. Bouret SG. Neurodevelopmental actions of leptin. Brain Res 2010;1350:2–9.

47. Udagawa J, Hatta T, Hashimoto R, et al. Roles of leptin in prenatal and perinatal brain development. Congenit Anom (Kyoto) 2007;47(3):77–83.

48. Piper K, Brickwood S, Turnpenny LW, et al. Beta cell differentiation during early human pancreas development. J Endocrinol 2004;181(1):11–23.

49. Heinze E, Steinke J. Insulin secretion during development: response of isolated pancreatic islets of fetal, newborn and adult rats to theophylline and arginine. Horm Metab Res 1972;4(4):234–6.

50. Mendonca AC, Carneiro EM, Bosqueiro JR, et al. Development of the insulin secretion mechanism in fetal and neonatal rat pancreatic B-cells: response to glucose, K+, theophylline, and carbamylcholine. Braz J Med Biol Res 1998;31(6):841–6.

51. Baumann MU, Deborde S, Illsley NP. Placental glucose transfer and fetal growth. Endocrine 2002;19(1):13–22.

52. Desoye G, Gauster M, Wadsack C. Placental transport in pregnancy pathologies. Am J Clin Nutr 2011;94(Suppl 6):1896S–902S.

53. Pedersen J. Diabetes mellitus and pregnancy: present status of the hyperglycaemia–hyperinsulinism theory and the weight of the newborn baby. Postgrad Med J 1971;(Suppl):66–7.

54. Pedersen J, Osler M. Hyperglycemia as the cause of characteristic features of the foetus and newborn of diabetic mothers. Dan Med Bull 1961;8:78–83.

55. Gauguier D, Bihoreau MT, Picon L, et al. Insulin secretion in adult rats after intrauterine exposure to mild hyperglycemia during late gestation. Diabetes 1991;40(Suppl 2):109–14.

56. Leloup C, Magnan C, Alquier T, et al. Intrauterine hyperglycemia increases insulin binding sites but not glucose transporter expression in discrete brain areas in term rat fetuses. Pediatr Res 2004;56(2):263–7.

57. Plagemann A, Harder T, Rake A, et al. Hypothalamic insulin and neuropeptide Y in the offspring of gestational diabetic mother rats. Neuroreport 1998;9(18):4069–73.

58. Plagemann A, Harder T, Janert U, et al. Malformations of hypothalamic nuclei in hyperinsulinemic offspring of rats with gestational diabetes. Dev Neurosci 1999;21(1):58–67.

59. Gupta A, Srinivasan M, Thamadilok S, et al. Hypothalamic alterations in fetuses of high fat diet-fed obese female rats. J Endocrinol 2009;200(3):293–300.

60. Pitkin RM, Van Orden DE. Fetal effects of maternal streptozotocin-diabetes. Endocrinology 1974;94(5):1247–53.

61. Chen H, Simar D, Lambert K, et al. Maternal and postnatal overnutrition differentially impact appetite regulators and fuel metabolism. Endocrinology 2008; 149(11):5348–56.
62. Kappy M, Sellinger S, Raizada M. Insulin binding in four regions of the developing rat brain. J Neurochem 1984;42(1):198–203.
63. Baron-Van Evercooren A, Olichon-Berthe C, Kowalski A, et al. Expression of IGF-I and insulin receptor genes in the rat central nervous system: a developmental, regional, and cellular analysis. J Neurosci Res 1991;28(2):244–53.
64. Brennan WA Jr. Developmental aspects of the rat brain insulin receptor: loss of sialic acid and fluctuation in number characterize fetal development. Endocrinology 1988;122(6):2364–70.
65. Ugrumov MV, Ivanova IP, Mitskevich MS. Permeability of the blood-brain barrier in the median eminence during the perinatal period in rats. Cell Tissue Res 1983; 230(3):649–60.
66. Singh BS, Westfall TC, Devaskar SU. Maternal diabetes-induced hyperglycemia and acute intracerebral hyperinsulinism suppress fetal brain neuropeptide Y concentrations. Endocrinology 1997;138(3):963–9.
67. Morris MJ, Chen H. Established maternal obesity in the rat reprograms hypothalamic appetite regulators and leptin signaling at birth. Int J Obes (Lond) 2009;33(1):115–22.
68. Carmody JS, Wan P, Accili D, et al. Respective contributions of maternal insulin resistance and diet to metabolic and hypothalamic phenotypes of progeny. Obesity (Silver Spring) 2011;19(3):492–9.
69. Steculorum SM, Bouret SG. Maternal diabetes compromises the organization of hypothalamic feeding circuits and impairs leptin sensitivity in offspring. Endocrinology 2011;152:4171–9.
70. Desai M, Li T, Ross MG. Fetal hypothalamic neuroprogenitor cell culture: preferential differentiation paths induced by leptin and insulin. Endocrinology 2011; 152(8):3192–201.
71. Plum L, Lin HV, Aizawa KS, et al. InsR/FoxO1 signaling curtails hypothalamic POMC neuron number. PLoS One 2012;7(2):e31487.
72. Plagemann A, Harder T, Rake A, et al. Increased number of galanin-neurons in the paraventricular hypothalamic nucleus of neonatally overfed weanling rats. Brain Res 1999;818(1):160–3.
73. Plagemann A, Harder T, Lindner R, et al. Alterations of hypothalamic catecholamines in the newborn offspring of gestational diabetic mother rats. Brain Res Dev Brain Res 1998;109(2):201–9.
74. Harder T, Franke K, Fahrenkrog S, et al. Prevention by maternal pancreatic islet transplantation of hypothalamic malformation in offspring of diabetic mother rats is already detectable at weaning. Neurosci Lett 2003;352(3):163–6.
75. Harder T, Aerts L, Franke K, et al. Pancreatic islet transplantation in diabetic pregnant rats prevents acquired malformation of the ventromedial hypothalamic nucleus in their offspring. Neurosci Lett 2001;299(1–2):85–8.
76. Franke K, Harder T, Aerts L, et al. 'Programming' of orexigenic and anorexigenic hypothalamic neurons in offspring of treated and untreated diabetic mother rats. Brain Res 2005;1031(2):276–83.
77. Fahrenkrog S, Harder T, Stolaczyk E, et al. Cross-fostering to diabetic rat dams affects early development of mediobasal hypothalamic nuclei regulating food intake, body weight, and metabolism. J Nutr 2004;134(3):648–54.
78. Schechter R, Abboud M, Johnson G. Brain endogenous insulin effects on neurite growth within fetal rat neuron cell cultures. Brain Res Dev Brain Res 1999;116(2): 159–67.

79. Toran-Allerand CD, Ellis L, Pfenninger KH. Estrogen and insulin synergism in neurite growth enhancement in vitro: mediation of steroid effects by interactions with growth factors? Brain Res 1988;469(1–2):87–100.
80. Harder T, Rake A, Rohde W, et al. Overweight and increased diabetes susceptibility in neonatally insulin-treated adult rats. Endocr Regul 1999;33(1):25–31.
81. Plagemann A, Heidrich I, Gotz F, et al. Lifelong enhanced diabetes susceptibility and obesity after temporary intrahypothalamic hyperinsulinism during brain organization. Exp Clin Endocrinol 1992;99(2):91–5.
82. Plagemann A, Harder T, Rake A, et al. Morphological alterations of hypothalamic nuclei due to intrahypothalamic hyperinsulinism in newborn rats. Int J Dev Neurosci 1999;17(1):37–44.
83. Kirk SL, Samuelsson AM, Argenton M, et al. Maternal obesity induced by diet in rats permanently influences central processes regulating food intake in offspring. PLoS One 2009;4(6):e5870.
84. Bouret SG, Gorski JN, Patterson CM, et al. Hypothalamic neural projections are permanently disrupted in diet-induced obese rats. Cell Metab 2008;7(2):179–85.
85. Lenz KM, McCarthy MM. Organized for sex - steroid hormones and the developing hypothalamus. Eur J Neurosci 2010;32(12):2096–104.
86. Simerly RB. Wired on hormones: endocrine regulation of hypothalamic development. Curr Opin Neurobiol 2005;15(1):81–5.
87. Heerwagen MJ, Miller MR, Barbour LA, et al. Maternal obesity and fetal metabolic programming: a fertile epigenetic soil. Am J Physiol Regul Integr Comp Physiol 2010;299(3):R711–22.
88. Davidowa H, Plagemann A. Insulin resistance of hypothalamic arcuate neurons in neonatally overfed rats. Neuroreport 2007;18(5):521–4.
89. Chen H, Morris MJ. Differential responses of orexigenic neuropeptides to fasting in offspring of obese mothers. Obesity (Silver Spring) 2009;17(7):1356–62.
90. Rother E, Kuschewski R, Alcazar MA, et al. Hypothalamic JNK1 and IKKbeta activation and impaired early postnatal glucose metabolism after maternal perinatal high-fat feeding. Endocrinology 2012;153(2):770–81.
91. Grayson BE, Levasseur PR, Williams SM, et al. Changes in melanocortin expression and inflammatory pathways in fetal offspring of nonhuman primates fed a high-fat diet. Endocrinology 2010;151(4):1622–32.
92. Dennery PA. Role of redox in fetal development and neonatal diseases. Antioxid Redox Signal 2004;6(1):147–53.
93. Dennery PA. Oxidative stress in development: nature or nurture? Free Radic Biol Med 2010;49(7):1147–51.
94. Kennedy KA, Sandiford SD, Skerjanc IS, et al. Reactive oxygen species and the neuronal fate. Cell Mol Life Sci 2012;69(2):215–21.
95. Koutcherov Y, Mai JK, Ashwell KW, et al. Organization of human hypothalamus in fetal development. J Comp Neurol 2002;446(4):301–24.
96. Chang GQ, Gaysinskaya V, Karatayev O, et al. Maternal high-fat diet and fetal programming: increased proliferation of hypothalamic peptide-producing neurons that increase risk for overeating and obesity. J Neurosci 2008;28(46):12107–19.
97. Rosenn BM, Miodovnik M. Glycemic control in the diabetic pregnancy: is tighter always better? J Matern Fetal Med 2000;9(1):29–34.
98. ter Braak EW, Evers IM, Willem Erkelens D, et al. Maternal hypoglycemia during pregnancy in type 1 diabetes: maternal and fetal consequences. Diabetes Metab Res Rev 2002;18(2):96–105.

Index

Note: Page numbers of article titles are in **boldface** type.

Endocrinol Metab Clin N Am 42 (2013) 165–186
http://dx.doi.org/10.1016/S0889-8529(12)00142-9
0889-8529/13/$ – see front matter © 2013 Elsevier Inc. All rights reserved.

endo.theclinics.com

Moving?

Make sure your subscription moves with you!

To notify us of your new address, find your **Clinics Account Number** (located on your mailing label above your name), and contact customer service at:

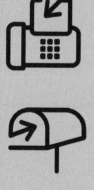

Email: journalscustomerservice-usa@elsevier.com

800-654-2452 (subscribers in the U.S. & Canada)
314-447-8871 (subscribers outside of the U.S. & Canada)

Fax number: 314-447-8029

Elsevier Health Sciences Division
Subscription Customer Service
3251 Riverport Lane
Maryland Heights, MO 63043

Printed and bound by CPI Group (UK) Ltd, Croydon, CR0 4YY

03/10/2024

01040442-0020